STUDY GUIDE

Kathy Demitrakis
Albuquerque Technical Vocational Institute

Donald Sharpe
University of Regina

SOCIAL PSYCHOLOGY

Second Canadian Edition

Elliot Aronson
University of Californis, Santa Cruz

Timothy D. Wilson
University of Virginia

Robin M. Akert
Wellesley College

Beverley Fehr
University of Winnipeg

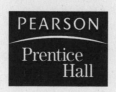

PEARSON
Prentice
Hall

Toronto

ISBN 0-13-121772-0

Executive Acquisitions Editor: Jessica Mosher
Senior Developmental Editor: Lise Dupont
Editorial Coordinator: Söğüt Y. Güleç
Production Manager: Wendy Moran

1 2 3 4 5   08 07 06 05 04

Printed and bound in Canada.

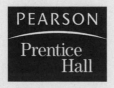

PEARSON
Prentice
Hall

TABLE OF CONTENTS

PREFACE TO THE STUDENT

Thanks for taking the time to look at this study guide. We hope that it assists you if you decide to use it for your psychology class. It is our hope that this supplement to your text will help you to study and to be better prepared to write exams and papers. We would like to take this opportunity to describe the sections that you will encounter in each chapter of this guide. We would also like to share some tips for using the guide and for maximizing your chances for success in your social psychology course.

The chapters begin with a *Chapter Overview* and a *Chapter Outline*. These are intended to provide you with a framework in which to fit in the details that you will discover in the textbook's chapters. Outlines are great learning tools as they help to organize material and make it easier to remember. We strongly suggest that you organize all of your study materials in this manner. You may want to add subheadings to the general outline. We encourage you to do this. If you make the material personally relevant, that will be a great asset to you in class.

The next section contains the *Learning Objectives* for the chapter. Use these both to instruct yourself regarding the important points in the text and to monitor your progress in a chapter. You may not be tested on all of these objectives, but using these to guide your reading and comprehension of the chapters will make you better prepared come exam time. The objectives are referenced by page numbers so if something sounds unfamiliar to you, you can refer to the text easily. The objectives are designed to give you a comprehensive guide to the chapters.

The *Key Terms* sections contain all of the terms that are given special attention in your textbook. We recommend that you learn these terms very well and that you look up any terms you can not easily recall. Most instructors consider knowledge of terminology to be vital to an understanding of the course. Try to do more than memorize the definitions of these terms, though. Apply them to your life (or to your friend's). You'll improve your chances of both remembering them for the test and of acquiring language to describe our social world to others.

The *Study Questions* sections are designed to help you answer essay questions on the topics in your textbook. They can also be helpful for stimulating paper topic ideas. We advise you to try to answer these questions even if you are taking only multiple choice exams in your class, because the answers will show you how the material is connected and applied. At the very least, read these questions over carefully and try to assess your ability to answer them effectively. Some space is provided for your answers. Feel free to use more space if you need it.

The last section consists of the *Practice Quiz* for the chapter. It enables you to test your knowledge of the chapter. Because testing yourself in different formats will make you more flexible for any exam format that you may face, we have included a variety of questions, including Fill-in-the-Blank, Multiple Choice, and Short Essay questions. One of the best ways to prepare for an exam is to take an exam. These quizzes will provide you with valuable practice for this class and for your other ones, too. All of the answers are supplied at the end of the study guide, and they are referenced by chapter and page to help you look up any material that you may need.

Finally, we wish you luck in your social psychology course! We sincerely hope that you will follow these suggestions and reap both academic and personal benefits from this study guide, your textbook, and your course.

Katherine M. Demitrakis

Donald Sharpe

CHAPTER 1

Introduction to Social Psychology

CHAPTER OVERVIEW

The first chapter is an introduction to the field and perspective of social psychology. A main focus of this chapter is to tell you what social psychology is and what it is not. In the first part of the chapter, you will discover similarities between social psychology and other disciplines, but note the important differences that set social psychology apart from fields that study similar phenomena. For example, it may be obvious why social psychology is different from folk wisdom, but distinguishing the perspective from personality psychology is more challenging. In the second part of the chapter, the important influences of the social situation on people's thoughts, feelings, and behaviours are stressed. This discussion helps to solidify social psychology's unique contribution to the study of social behaviour. To understand how the social psychological perspective got started, historical developments which include behaviourism and gestalt psychology are addressed in this section.

The third part of the chapter describes two fundamental approaches to the study of social behaviour. To master the rest of the text it is very important to know the basic assumptions of each approach. The application of social psychology to solving social problems is considered in the last part of the chapter.

CHAPTER OUTLINE

What is Social Psychology?

> Some Alternative Ways of Understanding Social Influence

> Social Psychology Compared to Sociology

> Social Psychology Compared to Personality Psychology

The Power of Social Influence

> Underestimating the Power of Social Influence

> The Subjectivity of the Social Situation

Where Construals Come From: Basic Human Motives

> The Self-Esteem Approach: The Desire to Feel Good About Ourselves

> The Social Cognition Approach: The Need to Be Accurate

> Other Motives: Ensuring Our Survival

1

LEARNING OBJECTIVES

After you have read Chapter 1, you should be able to do the following:

1. Define social psychology. Define social influence and state why it is of interest to social psychologists. Define *construals*. Indicate why social psychologists study these rather than simply the objective environments of people. (pp. 3-5)

2. Indicate how the approach taken by social psychologists is different from that of philosophers and social commentators. Describe why the social psychological approach may lead to more accurate predictions about human behaviour compared to the other approaches. (pp. 5-8)

3. Compare and contrast how sociology, personality psychology, and social psychology attempt to understand and predict human behaviour. Identify the goals of sociology compared to those of social psychology. Define the term individual differences. Identify the goals of personality psychology compared to those of social psychology. (pp. 8-10)

4. Define the term fundamental attribution error. Identify the consequences of making this error and underestimating the power of social influence. (pp. 10-13)

5. Explain how social psychology was influenced by Behaviourism and Gestalt psychology. Identify what each school of psychology has contributed to social psychology. (pp. 13-15)

6. Identify the two basic motives that underlie the origins of people's construals. Describe what happens when the two basic human motives conflict. (pp. 15-17)

7. Identify the approaches associated with the two basic human motives. Define the term self-esteem. Define the term social cognition. Describe the assumptions of each approach. (pp. 17-22)

8. Identify other motives that influence the formation of people's construals. What is evolutionary psychology? (pp. 22-23)

9. Identify some social problems that social psychologists research and attempt to remedy. (pp. 23-25)

KEY TERMS

social psychology (p. 4)

construal (p. 4)

individual differences (p. 9)

the fundamental attribution error (p. 10)

behaviourism (p. 13)

Gestalt psychology (p. 14)

self-esteem (p. 17)

social cognition (p. 20)

evolutionary psychology (p. 22)

STUDY QUESTIONS

1. What do social psychologists study scientifically?

   - how people's thots, feelings, behaviours are infl.
     by the real or imagined presence of others.

2. List examples of social influence.

   - direct persuasion
   - advertising.

3. What is contained in a person's construal of the world?

   - how people perceive, comprehend, & interpret the social world
   - interpretation!

4. Although they may share the same questions, what advantages does social psychology have over folk wisdom and philosophy in answering these questions?

   - no oversimplification, or underestimate power of the situation
   - address empirically, scientifically.

5. What do sociologists study?

6. Which branch of psychology studies how individual differences between people explain their behaviour?

7. What are some examples of individual differences?
   - bold vs. timid
   - selfish
   - conformist

8. What is the fundamental attribution error? Why do people commit this error when they try to explain other people's behaviour?
   - overestimating people's behaviour due to internal, dispositional factors & underestimating the role of situational factors.
   - experience false security, comforts us, blame victims

9. What are some consequences of committing the fundamental attribution error? - increases vulnerability to destructive social influence
   - make inaccurate predictions.

10. According to Behaviourism, what do we need to consider to understand human behaviour?
    - reinforcing properties of the env.

11. What has Gestalt psychology contributed to social psychology?
    (construal emph).
    - shud study the subj. way in which an object appears in people's minds.

12. List and define the two basic motives that help to form people's construals.
    - self-esteem; desire to feel good about ourselves
    - social cogn; need to be accurate.

13. Why do people engage in self-justification and what are some of its consequences?
    - to feel better about ourselves; decreases the probability to learn from experiences.
    - distort interpretation of reality.

14. What is an assumption of the social cognition approach? What interferes with the accuracy of this assumption?

    — that all people try to view the world as accurately as possible.
    — generally never know all the facts we need to make accurate judgements of a situation.

15. What is the relationship between people's motive to be accurate and their expectations about the social world? What can result from people's expectations?

    — can change the nature of the social world
    ⇒ "self-fulfilling prophecy"

PRACTICE QUIZ CHAPTER 1

Fill-in-the-blank

1. The scientific study of the way in which people's thoughts, feelings, and behaviours are influenced by the real or imagined presence of other people is called

   _____.

2. The effects of the real or imagined presence of others on people's thoughts, feelings, and behaviours is called _____.

3. The way in which people perceive, comprehend, and interpret the social world is their _____ of the world.

4. A social science concerned with topics such as social class, social structure, and social institutions is called

   _____.

5. Aspects of people's personalities that make them different from other people are called _____.

6. A discipline in psychology that focuses on individual differences as explanations of social behaviour is known as _____.

7. The tendency to overestimate the extent to which people's behaviour is due to internal, dispositional factors and to underestimate the role of situational factors is called the _____.

8. A school of psychology which says that human behaviour can be understood by examining the reinforcing properties of the environment is called

   _____.

9. A school of psychology that stresses the importance of studying the subjective way in which an object appears in people's minds, rather than the objective, physical attributes of the object is called _____.

10. The extent to which people view themselves as good, competent, and decent is called _____.

11. How people select, interpret, remember, and use social information is called _____.

12. A social psychological phenomenon whereby people's expectations evoke behaviour that confirms the expectations is called _____.

Multiple Choice

13. Social psychology is not concerned with social situations in any objective sense, but with how people are influenced by
    a) their construal of the social environment.
    b) abstract social rules and customs.
    c) social situations they've encountered in the past.
    d) their interactions with other people in social situations.

14. The major reason why we have conflicting folk aphorisms like "birds of a feather flock together" and "opposites attract" is that
    a) one of the sayings does not accurately describe human nature.
    b) for some people one saying applies while for others the opposite is applicable.
    c) there are some conditions under which one saying is correct and other conditions in which the opposite is true.
    d) such sayings were developed in different cultures that taught contrasting values.

15. Psychologists interested in the effects of different personality traits on aggressive behaviour are referred to as
    (a) personality psychologists.
    (b) social psychologists.
    (c) behaviourist psychologists.
    (d) Gestalt psychologists.

16. Why is it difficult for social psychologists to convince people that their behaviour is greatly influenced by the social environment?
    a) Because people outside of social psychology are rarely interested in the causes of social behaviour.
    b) Because people are motivated to perceive the world accurately.
    c) Because people are inclined to commit the fundamental attribution error in explaining behaviour.
    d) all of the above

17. Behavioural psychologists like Watson and Skinner believed that all human behaviour could be understood by examining
    a)   rewards and punishments in the individual's environment.
    b)   the impact of broad social and cultural factors on the individual.
    c)   how the individual thinks and feels about rewards and punishments.
    d)   how the individual is rewarded and punished for having various thoughts and feelings.

18. Research on hazing shows that members like a group better if they had endured unpleasant procedures to get into the group than if they had not. These findings are best accounted for by
    a)   self-justification.
    b)   the fundamental attribution error.
    c)   principles of reinforcement.
    d)   the self-fulfilling prophecy.

19. According to the social cognition approach,
    a)   people try to view the world as accurately as possible.
    b)   people do their best to understand and predict the social world.
    c)   coming up with an accurate picture of the social world is often difficult.
    d)   all of the above

20. Social psychologists are primarily concerned that their ideas about human social behaviour
    a)   withstand empirical testing.
    b)   obey philosophical principles.
    c)   adhere to conventional wisdom.
    d)   make sense intuitively.

21. Sociologists focus on _____ for explanations of human behaviour whereas social psychologists focus on _____ for such explanations.
    a)   society; the individual
    b)   society; people's past experiences
    c)   people's past experiences; the individual
    d)   the individual; society

22. When we commit the fundamental attribution error in explaining people's behaviour we _____ the power of personality traits and _____ the power of social influence.
    a)   overestimate; underestimate
    b)   overestimate; overestimate
    c)   underestimate; overestimate
    d)   underestimate; underestimate

23. By emphasising the way in which people construe the social world, social psychology has its direct roots more in the tradition of _____ than in behaviourism.
    a) sociology
    b) personality psychology
    c) developmental psychology
    d) Gestalt psychology

24. Whereas the _____ approach emphasises that behaviour is motivated by the desire to feel good about ourselves, the _____ approach emphasises the need to be accurate.
    a) self-esteem; rational
    b) emotional; rational
    c) social cognition; emotional
    d) self-esteem; social cognition

25. Researchers who attempt to understand social behaviour from the perspective of social cognition assume that we
    a) have a limitless capacity to process information.
    b) try to view the world as accurately as possible.
    c) logically suspend our judgements until we have gathered all the relevant facts.
    d) are primarily motivated to view ourselves as rational.

26. You expect that people at a party will not enjoy your company. Consequently, you spare them the misery of talking with you by being brief and cutting short their conversations with you. Later you learn that your company was not enjoyed. What social psychological phenomenon has occurred in this situation?
    a) social cognition
    b) self-justification
    c) reinforcement
    d) self-fulfilling prophesy

27. Social psychologists attempting to convince people to conserve natural resources will first
    a) delineate the rewards and punishments in the situation which block conservation efforts.
    b) increase people's awareness that natural resources need to be conserved.
    c) identify the motives underlying people's failure to conserve.
    d) adopt a "let's wait and see" approach to the problem of conservation.

Short Essay

28. Linda, a social psychologist, and Mark, a sociologist, take a walk in a park where they witness a fight between two youths. What explanations are Linda and Mark likely to offer for the aggressive behaviour they observed?

29. Compare the self-esteem and social cognition approaches to the study of social behaviour. What assumptions are made by each approach?

30. What is the critical distinction between social psychology and folk wisdom philosophy? What is the advantage of social psychology's approach to social behaviour?

31. Describe an instance of the self-fulfilling prophecy from your own experiences.

32. Discuss ways in which you are influenced by both the real and imagined presence of others.

CHAPTER 2

Methodology: How Social Psychologists Do Research

CHAPTER OVERVIEW

Chapter 2 contains the basic underlying principles of social psychological research. Some of the material may sound familiar to you, however, it is vital to know the concepts in this chapter well. A firm understanding of this material will increase the enjoyment you receive from reading the rest of the text. Mastery of these concepts will also help you be more critical of research findings you read in the text and those you are exposed to in the media.

The first part of the chapter introduces you to the beginning of the research process, the formation of theories and hypotheses. The next part discusses the types, advantages, and disadvantages of descriptive methods. In the next section, the experimental method is described. This section contains perhaps the most technical information in the chapter. It is recommended that you learn both definitions and applications of the basic components of this method. Remember that although conclusions about causality may be derived only from experiments, the method used depends on the particular research question being asked. Keep in mind the goals of each type of method as you read about each of them. In the next section of this chapter, ethical issues in social psychology are discussed. Psychological researchers must abide by strict guidelines to insure the welfare of participants in their research. Due to the phenomena that some social psychologists study, ethical research in the field may involve a strong element of creativity. Basic and applied research are compared in the last section.

CHAPTER OUTLINE

Social Psychology: An Empirical Science

Formulating Hypotheses and Theories

Descriptive Methods: Describing Social Behaviour

      The Observational Method

      Archival Analysis

      The Correlational Method

The Experimental Method: Answering Causal Questions

      Independent and Dependent Variables

      Internal Validity in Experiments

External Validity in Experiments

The Basic Dilemma of the Experimental Social Psychologist

Ethical Issues in Social Psychology

Basic Versus Applied Research

LEARNING OBJECTIVES

After you read Chapter 2, you should be able to do the following:

1. Explain why social psychological results sometimes appear obvious. (pp. 30-32)

2. Explain why it is necessary to translate beliefs into hypotheses. Describe the process of theory refinement. (pp. 32-34)

3. Identify the goal of the observational method and distinguish between everyday observations and systematic observations. Describe participant observation and define interjudge reliability (pp. 34-37)

4. Describe the procedures used in archival analysis. (pp. 37-39)

5. Identify the goal of the correlational method. Discuss and define the characteristics of a correlation. Define and state possible values of a positive correlation. Define and state possible values of a negative correlation. (pp. 39-40)

6. Identify the role of surveys and samples in conducting correlational research. Explain the importance of selecting samples randomly. Identify potential threats to obtaining inaccurate survey results. Define random selection. (pp. 40-42)

7. Distinguish between correlation and causation. Identify three possible causal relationships between variables that are correlated. (pp. 42-44)

8. Identify the goal and components of the experimental method. (pp. 44-47)

9. Distinguish between independent and dependent variables. (p. 47)

10. Define internal validity. Identify factors that threaten the internal validity of an experiment. Define random assignment to conditions and explain why it is necessary to internal validity. Define the term probability value and explain what a p-value tells us. Describe the conditions under which results are considered statistically significant. (pp. 48-49)

11.   Define external validity. Identify the kinds of generalisability that concern researchers. What is the connection between meta-analysis and replication? Define mundane realism and psychological realism. (pp. 49-52)

12.   Describe the basic dilemma of the social psychologist. Compare and contrast lab experiments and field experiments. Describe the relationship between internal and external validity and each type of experimental setting. (pp. 53-54)

13.   Describe the ethical dilemma faced by social psychologists and the role of informed consent in resolving this dilemma.   Identify a deception experiment. Explain the necessity and functions of a debriefing session. Discuss the effects on participants of being deceived. (pp. 55-57)

14.   Contrast the goals of basic and applied research. Discuss the relationship between these types of research. (pp. 57-59)

KEY TERMS

theory (p. 32)

observational method (p. 35)

operational definition (p. 36)

participant observation (p. 36)

interjudge reliability (p. 37)

archival analysis (p. 37)

correlational method (p. 39)

correlation coefficient (p. 39)

surveys (p. 40)

random selection (p. 40)

experimental method (p. 44)

independent variable (p. 47)

dependent variable (p. 47)

random assignment to condition (p. 48)

probability level (p-value) (p. 48)

internal validity (p. 49)

external validity (p. 49)

mundane realism (p. 49)

psychological realism (p. 50)

cover story (p. 50)

replication (p. 51)

meta-analysis (p. 51)

field experiments (p. 53)

informed consent (p. 55)

deception (p. 55)

debriefing (p. 56)

basic research (p. 58)

applied research (p. 58)

STUDY QUESTIONS

1.   Why do some conclusions about social behaviour seem obvious?

     – topic = intimately familiar: social behaviour & social influence.

2.   How are theories and hypotheses formulated?

     – dissatisfaction w/existing theories & explanations, previous research,
        observations of everyday life ⇒ construct a theory, design a study to test
     – collect data to test hypothesis

3.   When would it be appropriate to conduct an archival analysis?

     – to measure behaviours that change over time, or across diff. cultures.

4.   Why is interjudge reliability necessary in observational studies?

     – to ensure observations are not the subjective impressions of one individual

5.   In addition to describing a relationship between two variables, what do
     correlations allow us to do?

     – assess how well can predict one variable based on another (correlation
        coefficient)

6.   What is a correlation coefficient? What does it tell us?

— statistical technique that assesses how well can predict one variable based on another

7.   What are some criteria for survey data collection in order to help insure that the data are accurate?

— random selection
— straightforward Q's

8.   What are the necessary components of an experiment?

— random assignment to conditions
— internal/external validity

9.   Regarding an experiment, what does high internal validity imply?

— ensuring that nothing other than the i.v. can affect the d.v. (by controlling all extraneous variables & randomly assigning people to diff. conditions)

10.   If a researcher used random assignment to conditions and found differences in the dependent variable across conditions, what may account for these differences?

— the i.v.

11.   Why might lab experiments lack external validity?

— lack of mundane realism (not similar to real-life situations)

12.   What is a meta analysis? What does it tell us about research findings?

— avgs. of results of 2 or more studies to see if effect of i.v. is reliable

13.   How do replications and cross-cultural research help to increase the external validity of research findings?

— more evidence for hypothesis if results same for studies w/ diff. subject populations or in diff. settings. ⟹ universal psych. processes / diffs. in psych processes (cultural infl.)

14.   What is a trade-off between lab and field experiments? Why are lab experiments conducted in social psychology? — internal & external validity.

— control, random assignment

15. What are the goals of basic research and how do they differ from those of applied research?

— to explain behaviour (intellectual curiosity) vs. attempting to solve specific social or psyc. problem.

16. Why is informed consent necessary but sometimes not feasible in social psychological research? What must be done when deception is used in an experiment? *— deception studies — debriefing*

PRACTICE QUIZ CHAPTER 2

Fill-in-the-blank

1. A form of the systematic observational method used by observers who interact with the people being observed is called _____.

2. A form of the observational method used by researchers who examine the accumulated documents of a culture is called _____.

3. The level of agreement between two or more people who independently observe and code a set of data is called _____.

4. The method of research whereby two or more variables are systematically measured and the relationships between them are assessed is called the _____.

5. A statistic that tells us how well we can predict one variable from another is called a _____.

6. A way of selecting a sample of people from a larger population so that everyone in the population has an equal chance of being selected is called _____.

7. A method whereby under controlled conditions the researcher randomly assigns participants to different conditions, varies a single aspect between these conditions, and measures behaviour is called the _____.

8. The variable that is manipulated to determine if it causes changes in another variable is called the _____.

9. The variable that is measured to determine whether it is influenced when another variable is manipulated is called the _____.

10. When the only aspect that varies between experimental conditions is the independent variable, an experiment is said to have _____.

11. The procedure which assures that all participants have an equal chance of taking part in any condition of an experiment is called _____.

12. A number, calculated with statistical techniques, which indicates the likelihood that the results of an experiment occurred by chance and were not due to the independent variable, is called the _____.

13. The extent to which the results of a study can be generalised to other situations and to other people is known as _____.

14. The extent to which an experiment captures psychological processes like those that occur in everyday life is called _____.

15. A study repeated again, often with different subject populations or in different settings, is called a(n) _____.

16. A statistical technique which allows researchers to assess the strength of the effects of the independent variable by looking at its effects over many replications is called _____.

17. An experiment that is conducted in a real-life setting is called a _____.

18. Research conducted to solve a particular social problem is known as
_____.

19. An individual's willingness to participate in an experiment after receiving a description of the kinds of experiences that participants will go through is called
_____.

20. Misleading or concealing from participants the true purpose of the study or the events that will actually transpire is called _____.

21. Explaining to participants, at the end of an experiment, the purpose of the study and exactly what transpired is called _____.

Multiple Choice

22. From dissonance theory, Leon Festinger was able to make specific predictions about when and how people would change their attitudes. We call these specific predictions
    a)   theories.
    b)   hypotheses.
    c)   observations.
    d)   methods.

23. Using archival analyses, scientists describe a culture by
    a)   surveying a representative sample of members in a culture.
    b)   observing the behaviour of members in a culture.
    c)   manipulating archives and measuring subsequent responses.
    d)   examining documents like magazines, diaries, and suicide notes.

24. When INCREASES in the value of one variable are associated with DECREASES in the value of the other variable, then the variables are
    a) positively correlated.
    b) negatively correlated.
    c) uncorrelated.
    d) independent.

25. As long as the sample is selected randomly, we can assume that the sampled responses
    a) are a reasonable match to responses of the whole population.
    b) correlate with one another.
    c) reflect the true beliefs and opinions of the individuals sampled.
    d) are determined by chance factors.

26. From studies which indicate that viewing television violence is correlated with aggressive behaviour in children, we can conclude that
    a) watching violence on television may cause aggressive behaviour.
    b) the aggressive personalities of some children may cause them to prefer violence on television.
    c) some third factor like a hostile home environment may cause some children to both prefer violence on television and to behave aggressively.
    d) all of the above are possible causal relationships.

27. A "_____ experiment" is similar in design to a laboratory experiment except that it is conducted in a natural setting.
    a) savannah
    b) field
    c) bush
    d) real-life

28. How should research be conducted in order to resolve the basic dilemma of the social psychologist?
    a) By doing replications, conduct some experiments that have internal validity and others that have external validity.
    b) Conduct carefully designed experiments that have both internal and external validity.
    c) Do all research in the field.
    d) Conduct applied rather than basic research.

29. Which of the following is a statistical technique that allows researchers to test how reliable the effects of an independent variable are over many replications?
    a) correlation coefficient
    b) deception
    c) meta analysis
    d) double blind

30. Two individuals independently observe the same behaviour at a playground. If one reports seven instances of "aggression" and the other records seventeen such instances, then _____ will be low.
    a) interjudge reliability
    b) internal validity
    c) generalizability
    d) external validity

31. If you found the correlation coefficient between height and weight to be +.74, you could conclude that
    a) you made a mistake in your calculations.
    b) as height increases, weight increases.
    c) as height increases, weight decreases.
    d) height and weight are uncorrelated.

32. Latane and Darley (1968) varied the number of witnesses to an emergency and measured helping behaviour. In this experiment _____ was the independent variable and _____ was the dependent variable.
    a) helping behaviour; the number of witnesses
    b) the number of witnesses; helping behaviour
    c) the emergency; helping behaviour
    d) number of witnesses; the emergency

33. When the only aspect that varies across conditions in an experiment is the independent variable(s), the experiment is said to have _____.
    a) internal validity
    b) external validity
    c) reliability
    d) generalizability

34. Social psychologists are most concerned with generalizability across
    a) independent and dependent variables.
    b) theories and hypotheses.
    c) identical experiments.
    d) situations and people.

35. In an experiment on how anonymity affects aggression (Zimbardo, 1970), participants wore bags on their heads and administered shocks to a victim in another room. Assuming that wearing bags gave participants a sense of anonymity, this procedure
    a) had mundane realism but not psychological realism.
    b) had psychological realism but not mundane realism.
    c) had both mundane realism and psychological realism.
    d) lacked both mundane realism and psychological realism.

36. The basic dilemma of the social psychologist is that
    a) there is usually a tradeoff in experiments between internal and external validity.
    b) individual differences among participants can never be ruled out as alternative explanations for experimental results.
    c) there is a tradeoff between mundane and psychological realism.
    d) people behave differently when they are being observed.

37. While ____ research aims to solve a specific problem, ____ research tries to understand human social behaviour purely for reasons of intellectual curiosity.
    a) basic; applied
    b) applied; basic
    c) theoretical; practical
    d) practical; theoretical

Short Essay

38. What kinds of behaviours do observational methods best assess? What questions are addressed by the use of the observational method?

39. A local news program asks viewers to place a 50 cent call to the station in order to survey opinions on gun control. Near the end of the program a reporter announces "Our survey results indicate that community members overwhelmingly support gun control." Why should you be sceptical about the conclusion drawn?

40. Why must the independent variable be the only thing that varies between the groups in an experiment?

41. What is the primary limitation of carefully controlled laboratory experiments and how can this limitation be overcome?

42. Under what conditions can deception experiments be conducted, and what procedures must be followed if deception is used?

CHAPTER 3

Social Cognition: How We Think About the Social World

CHAPTER OVERVIEW

Chapter 3 informs us of the procedures, strategies, and problems we exhibit when we perceive and judge the social world. A main theme of this chapter concerns the biases that may colour our perceptions and judgements of others. The major influence of schemas on the processing of information about the social world is addressed in the first section of the chapter. Other mental shortcuts we use to conserve cognitive resources are also examined. Examples of judgmental heuristics (availability, representativeness, anchoring and adjustment, etc.) and the functions and problems associated with their use is a significant topic of this section.

The chapter also describes the distinction between automatic and controlled thinking. This distinction helps explain the flexibility of the social thinker. The effects of motivation and cognitive load figure prominently on our ability to be accurate perceivers and judges. The last section of the chapter tells us about the utility of teaching people to improve their reasoning skills. Educating people about the errors that are characteristic of our thinking has proven useful in the goal of improving people's perceptions and judgements of others.

CHAPTER OVERVIEW

People as Everyday Theorists: Schemas and their Influence

      The Function of Schemas: Why do We Have Them?

      Why Schemas are Applied? Accessibility and Priming.

      Schemas Can Persist Even After They Are Discredited

      Making Our Schemas Come True: The Self-Fulfilling Prophecy

      Cultural Determinants of Schemas

Mental Strategies and Shortcuts: Heuristics

      How Easily Does It Come to Mind? The Availability Heuristic

      How Similar Is A to B? The Representativeness Heuristic

      Taking Things at Face Value: The Anchoring and Adjustment Heuristic

Automatic versus Controlled Thinking

      Thought Suppression

      Thinking about What Might Have Been: Counterfactual Reasoning

A Portrayal of Social Thinking

Improving Human Thinking

LEARNING OBJECTIVES

After reading Chapter 3, you should be able to do the following:

1. Define a schema. Discuss its effects on attention, interpretation, and memory. (pp. 63-65)

2. Identify the functions of schemas. Describe conditions when schemas are very important.
(pp. 65-67)

3. Describe the role of accessibility and priming in our schema selection. (pp. 67-69)
   - recent exp. (arbitrary) = priming

4. How can schemas persist even after they are discredited? Describe the role of perseverance effects. (pp. 69-71)

5. Explain how the self-fulfilling prophecy makes schemas resistant to change. (pp. 71-73)

6. Describe the relationship between schemas and culture. (pp. 73-75)

7. Define judgmental heuristics and the advantages and limitations of using these heuristics. (pp. 75-76)

8. Define the availability heuristic. Discuss reasons why the availability heuristic may result in faulty judgements. Identify conditions that increase the availability of information in memory. (pp. 76-79)

9. Define the representativeness heuristic. Define base rate information. Discuss why the use of the representativeness heuristic results in the underuse of base rate information. (pp. 80-81)

10. Describe the process by which anchoring and adjustment are used to make judgements. Define the anchoring and adjustment heuristic and the consequences of its use. Define biased sampling. Describe the consequences of generalising information from a biased sample to the population. (pp. 81-85)

11. Identify the characteristics of automatic and controlled processing. Describe Gilbert's model of automatic believing and how it relates to automatic and controlled processing. (pp. 85-87) auto: Initially accept info   Controlled: assess truthfulness → unaccept if necessary.

12. Describe the two-part process involved in successful thought suppression. (pp. 87-89)

auto: monitoring process   Controlled: operating process
(conscious attempt to distract)

13. Define counterfactual thinking. Discuss conditions that facilitate counterfactual thinking. (pp. 90-93)

14. Define the overconfidence barrier. Discuss the effectiveness of teaching people basic statistical and methodological reasoning principles. (pp. 93-95)

KEY TERMS

social cognition (p. 63)

schemas (p. 63)

accessibility (p. 67)

priming (p. 68)

perseverance effect (p. 71)

self-fulfilling prophecy (p. 71)

judgmental heuristics (p. 76)

availability heuristic (p. 77)

availability (p. 77)

representativeness heuristic (p. 80)

base rate information (p. 80)

anchoring and adjustment heuristic (p. 81)

biased sampling (p. 82)

automatic processing (p. 85)

controlled processing (p. 85)

thought suppression (p. 87)

counterfactual thinking (p. 90)

overconfidence barrier (p. 94)

STUDY QUESTIONS

1. What is social cognition? What do researchers in this area study?

   — how people think about themselves & the social world — how people select, interpret, remember & use social info to make judgements & decisions

   — the procedures, rules & strategies people use: schemas, heuristics etc.

2. Why are schemas so important to study? What role do they play in people's understanding and interpretations of themselves and the social world? What are examples of cognitive processes that are influenced by schemas?

   — affect what info one notices, thinks about & remembers.

3. What functions do schemas serve? Why does their use sometimes have adaptive value? How is their use maladaptive?

   — for continuity; to relate new experiences to past schemas; reduce amt. of info needed to process; reduces ambiguity.

4. Why does the self-fulfilling prophecy occur? What function does it serve? How can it affect resistance to schema change?

   — by having expectations of others

5. Why do people use judgmental heuristics? What are three heuristics that people use to make judgements? When people rely on these heuristics what kind of information are they not taking into account?

   — mental shortcuts to make judgements quickly & efficiently.

   — availability heuristic; representativeness heuristic; anchoring & adjustment heuristic.

6. What is the relationship between the occurrence of counterfactual thinking and emotional reactions to events?

   — outcomes better than reality = "upward counterfactuals" → can serve a preparative function for the future (but more distressing)

   — outcomes worse than reality = downward counterfactuals" → help us feel better.

7. What are the advantages of automatic processing? When is automatic processing problematic?

   — allows us to think/perform efficiently

   — "seeing is believing" (Gilbert's Theory), takes effort/motivation to unaccept everything.

8. How do automatic processing and controlled processing interact to allow for successful thought suppression?

   monitoring process/ operating process

9. What can we teach people so that they overcome the overconfidence barrier and become better reasoners?

— when people have too much confidence in the accuracy of their judgements.

PRACTICE QUIZ CHAPTER 3

Fill-in-the-Blank

1. Cognitive structures people have to organise their knowledge about the social world by themes or subjects are called _____.

2. Mentally changing some part of the past to imagine what might have been is called. _____.

3. The persistence of people's beliefs after evidence supporting these beliefs has been discredited is called the _____.

4. An expectation about what another person is like which influences how one acts toward that person and causes that person to behave in a way that is consistent with the expectation is called a(n) _____.

5. Mental shortcuts people use to make judgements quickly and efficiently are called _____.

6. A heuristic whereby judgements are based on the ease with which something can be brought to mind is called the _____.

7. A heuristic whereby things are classified according to how similar they are to a typical case is called the _____.

8. Information about the frequency of members of different categories in the population is called _____.

9. A heuristic whereby judgements are made by adjusting an answer away from an initial value is called the _____.

10. Making generalizations from samples of information known to be a biased or atypical is called _____.

11. The finding that people usually have too much confidence in the accuracy of their own judgements has been labelled the _____.

12. The extent to which schemas are likely to be used when making judgments because they are at the forefront of people's minds is called _____.

13. A recent experience that increases a schema's accessibility is called

_____.

14. Thinking that is non-conscious, unintentional, involuntary, and effortless is called

_____.

Multiple Choice

15. We are most likely to use schemas to "fill in the blanks" when we
   a)   observe uninteresting stimuli.
   b)   observe familiar stimuli.
   c)   are uncertain what it is that we're observing.
   d)   fail to attend to what we are observing.

16. People's beliefs about themselves and the social world persist even after the evidence supporting their beliefs is discredited. This finding has been labelled the
   a)   persistence problem.
   b)   perseverance effect.
   c)   self-fulfilling prophesy.
   d)   overconfidence barrier.

17. The self-fulfilling prophecy makes schemas resistant to change because
   a)   it distorts our perceptions of disconfirming evidence.
   b)   it produces the evidence the individual needs to confirm the schema.
   c)   it provides a theme or topic around which a schema can be structured.
   d)   all of the above

18. When we base our judgements on the ease with which we can bring something to mind, we are using the _____ heuristic.
   a)   availability
   b)   representativeness
   c)   anchoring/adjustment
   d)   retrievability

19. Given information about a specific person which contradicts base rate information, people tend to
   a)   ignore the information about the person and use only the base rate information.
   b)   integrate the information about the individual and the base rate information.
   c)   look for another heuristic.
   d)   ignore the base rate, judging only how representative the information about the person is of a general category.

20. Which of the following is most likely performed using controlled processing?
   a)   tying one's shoes
   b)   calculating the answer to a difficult math problem
   c)   walking around one's house
   d)   using established stereotypes to form an impression of someone

21. Because people think that their reasoning processes are less fallible than they actually are, anyone trying to improve people's accuracy is up against a(n) _____.
    a) certainty threshold
    b) perseverance effect
    c) illusory correlation
    d) overconfidence barrier

22. Kelley (1950) had students read different descriptions of a guest lecturer who they evaluated at the end of class. Results indicated that
    a) the descriptions influenced how students rated the lecturer's unambiguous behaviours.
    b) the descriptions influenced students to such an extent that they failed to differentiate between ambiguous and unambiguous behaviours.
    c) the descriptions had no effect on the students' ratings.
    d) the descriptions influenced how students rated the lecturer's ambiguous behaviours.

23. Which of the following is NOT an advantage of viewing the world through schema-tinted glasses?
    a) Schemas allow us to interpret the meaning of ambiguous behaviour.
    b) Schemas facilitate the unbiased processing of information.
    c) Schemas facilitate smooth social interactions.
    d) Schemas allow us to deal with experiences in a manner that requires little cognitive effort.

24. Any time people act on their schemas in such a way that makes the schema "come true," a(n) _____ results.
    a) stereotype
    b) self-fulfilling prophesy
    c) illusory correlation
    d) perseverance effect

25. Making judgements by comparing someone to a stereotype demonstrates the use of a(n) _____ heuristic.
    a) anchoring
    b) representative
    c) adjustment
    d) unavailable

26. Which is NOT a characteristic of counterfactual thinking?
    a) it decreases the strength of emotional reactions to a negative event
    b) it increases the strength of emotional reactions to a negative event
    c) it occurs in response to an unexpected outcome
    d) its likelihood is influenced by the ease of mentally undoing an actual outcome

27. Processing that is conscious, intentional, voluntary, and effortful is called
    a) automatic
    b) controlled
    c) priming
    d) availability

28. Sullivan and colleagues (1997) asked students not to think about immersing their hands in ice-water for nine minutes. Compared to students asked simply to record their thoughts, the thought suppression students
    a) rated the ice-water immersion as less painful
    b) reported thoughts such as "I wonder if it will hurt"
    c) engaged in active coping strategies
    d) refused to participate in the immersion task

29. If you were in a minor car accident but imagined that the accident was worse than it was, Roese and Olson (1997) would suggest you are engaging in
    a) downward counterfactuals
    b) upward counterfactuals
    c) self-fulfilling prophecy
    d) automatic thinking

Short Essay

30. Describe three heuristics that aid our judgements. Give examples of each one.

31. What approach has been demonstrated to reduce people's overconfidence. The effectiveness of this approach suggests that overconfidence results from what?

32. Describe the influence of culture on the content of schemas.

33. Contrast automatic and controlled processing. Describe how these processes are involved in thought suppression.

34. Amy's taking out an ad in the classified to sell her old car. She knows that if she prints "Make offer" that people will offer her about $2000 for the car. Instead, she prints "$3000 or best offer." Why might she expect to receive higher bids for her car using this strategy?

35. You have noticed that a friend of yours seems especially prone to jump to conclusions about people on the basis of very little information about them. Naturally, you suspect that he/she is committing errors in inference. Using what you learned in Chapter 3, describe how you would attempt to correct your friend's errors.

CHAPTER 4

Social Perception: How We Come to Understand Other People

CHAPTER OVERVIEW

The topic of Chapter 4 is how we attempt to understand and explain the behaviours of others. The first section of the chapter depicts the ability we have to decode and encode nonverbal behaviour. In the next section we see that we use implicit personality theories to understand other people.

The third section consists of various models in the area of attribution theory. Causal attributions are reasons we formulate to explain the behaviour of others. Social psychologists have proposed several attribution theories. The covariation model focuses on how we make internal (personality) attributions to explain other people's behaviours. The attributional process does not always yield accurate attributions for both others and our own behaviours. Why these errors occur is discussed. The final section of this chapter addresses the accuracy of our attributions and impressions. Like our other perceptions of the social world, our perceptions of others may be somewhat inaccurate. Our preconceptions of other people can have a powerful influence on their behaviour and the perpetuation of the behaviours we expect can be realised.

CHAPTER OUTLINE

Nonverbal Behaviour

      Facial Expressions of Emotion

      Other Channels of Nonverbal Communication

Implicit Personality Theories: Filling in the Blanks

Causal Attribution: Answering the "Why" Question

      The Nature of the Attributional Process

      The Covariation Model: Internal Versus External Attributions

      The Fundamental Attribution Error: People as Personality Psychologists

      The Actor/Observer Difference

      Self-serving Attributions

      Blaming the Victim: An Unfortunate By-product of Attributional Processes

How Accurate Are Our Attributions and Impressions?

LEARNING OBJECTIVES

After reading Chapter 4, you should be able to do the following:

1. Define social perception. (p. 100)

2. Identify the various functions of nonverbal behaviour. (pp. 100-101)

3. Discuss universal facial expressions of emotion and research that supports this theory. (pp. 101-105)

4. Define affect blend and display rules. List examples of cross-cultural differences in nonverbal communication. (pp. 105-106)

5. Discuss other channels of nonverbal communication and define emblems. (pp. 106-108)

6. Define and discuss the origins, functions, and drawbacks of implicit personality theories. Discuss cross-cultural differences in the content of implicit personality theories. (pp. 108-111)

7. Identify the focus of attribution theory. Describe the nature of the attributional process according to Fritz Heider. Distinguish between internal and external attributions. (pp. 111-113)

8. Describe the covariation model of Kelley and the process it attempts to describe. Identify and define the three kinds of information Kelley claims we use to make attributions. Identify the types of attributions we make when these kinds of information are used together. (pp. 113-115)

9. Define the fundamental attribution error. Discuss why the fundamental attribution error is so prevalent. Discuss why it is called "fundamental." (pp. 115-117)

10. Discuss the role of perceptual salience in creating the fundamental attribution error. (pp. 117-119)

11. Discuss cross-cultural differences in the prevalence of the fundamental attribution error. (pp. 119-121)

12. Define the actor/observer difference and its relationship to the fundamental attribution error. Discuss the causes of the actor/observer difference. Identify the influences of perceptual salience and information availability on the actor/observer difference. (pp. 121-124)

13. Identify self-serving attributions for success and for failure. Discuss why people make self-serving attributions. (pp. 124-127)

14. Discuss the motives underlying defensive attributions. Identify and define two forms of defensive attributions. (pp. 127-129)

15. Discuss the "blaming the victim" of misfortune. Define the belief in a just world. (pp. 129-133)

16. Discuss the accuracy of our attributions and impressions of strangers and friends. Explain why our impressions of others are sometimes wrong and why we might not realise it. (pp. 133-135)

KEY TERMS

social perception (p. 100)

nonverbal communication (p. 100)

encode (p. 101)

decode (p. 101)

affect blend (p. 105)

display rules (p. 105)

emblems (p. 108)

implicit personality theory (p. 108)

attribution theory (p. 111)

internal attribution (p. 111)

external attribution (p. 111)

covariation model (p. 113)

consensus information (p. 113)

distinctiveness information (p. 113)

consistency information (p. 113)

fundamental attribution error (p. 116)

perceptual salience (p. 118)

actor/observer difference (p. 121)

self-serving attributions (p. 124)

defensive attributions (p. 127)

STUDY QUESTIONS

1. What are the most often used and diagnostic channels of nonverbal communication? What are other channels of nonverbal communication? What functions do nonverbal cues serve?

    - facial expressions
    - eye contact/gaze; personal space; gestures (emblems)
    - express (encode) emotion, convey attitudes, communicate personality traits, facilitate/regulate verbal speech.

2. What is the relationship between encoding and decoding? What are the six major emotional expressions that are universally encoded and decoded?

    - expressing/emitting verbal codes vs. interpreting meaning of verbal codes.
    - anger, happiness, fear, surprise, sadness, disgust (contempt?)

3. What are display rules? What are examples of cross-cultural differences in display rules?

    - culturally determined rules about which non-verbal behaviours are appropriate to display.

4. What are affect blends? What are emblems? What are examples of both of these?

    - a facial expression that registers more than one emotion (on diff. parts of face).
    - nonverbal gestures, w/well-understood cultural defns. (usu. direct verbal translations)

5. Who may be better at decoding nonverbal cues, extroverts or introverts, men or women?

6. What is an implicit personality theory? What are functions of implicit personality theories?

    - type of schema that groups various personality traits together, to fill-in-the-blanks about impression of other people.

7. What is attribution theory? What does it try to describe and explain? How do internal attributions differ from external ones?

    - description of the way people explain the causes of people's behaviours
    - internal = dispositional/personality vs. external = situational.

8. What are the two types of social expectancies that influence attribution formation?

- people generally prefer internal attributions over external ones
  - we generally focus/notice people & their behaviour/not the situation.

9. What is the premise of the covariation model? What information do we examine for covariation when we form attributions? When are people most likely to make an internal attribution and an external attribution according to the covariation model? — how people decide to make an internal vs external attribution by noting the pattern between the presence or absence of possible causal factors ⇒ consensus, distinctiveness, consistency.
  - external attribution if all high; internal if low/low/high consistency

10. What is the fundamental attribution error? Why does it occur? What is perceptual salience? What are cross-cultural differences in the rate of the fundamental attribution error? — tendency to overestimate people's internal dispositional factors & underestimate the role of situational factors.
  - our focus usu. on one's behaviour, not the situation, usu. invisible to us = perceptual salience ⇒ usu. overestimate causal role of perceptually salient info.

11. What is the actor/observer difference? Why does it occur?
  - tendency to see others' behaviour as dispositionally caused & our own behaviour as situational (b/c perceptual salience, info availability).
  West = prefer dispositional outlook
  East = prefer situational explanations

12. When we form self-serving attributions to what do we attribute our successes and our failures?
  - successes = dispositional factors; failures = situational factors.

13. What are defensive attributions? What is unrealistic optimism? What is the belief in a just world? What functions do these defensive attributions serve?
  - explanations for behaviour that avoid feelings of vulnerability/mortality.
  - "U.O" = defensive attr. where people think good things more likely to happen to them & bad things less likely. - "B.I.A J.W." = people assume bad things happen to bad people, good things happen to good people.

14. What are some reasons why our impressions of others are sometimes incorrect? Why don't we know when our impressions of others are wrong?
  - fundamental attr. error ⇒ focus more on personalities vs. situation.
  - use of schemas; implicit personality theory
  - self-fulfilling prophecies.
  - to build self-esteem, make ourselves feel better.

PRACTICE QUIZ CHAPTER 4

Fill-in-the-blank

1. The study of how we form impressions of and make inferences about other people is called _____.

2. Research that studies how people communicate without spoken language is called
    _____.

3. To _____ is to express emotions and to _____ is to interpret them.

4. Culturally determined rules about the nonverbal behaviours that are appropriate to
    display are called _____.

5. Facial expressions where parts of the face are displaying different emotions are referred
    to as _____.

6. Nonverbal gestures that have clear, well-understood definitions within a given culture
    are called _____.

7. Schemas that people use to group various kinds of personality traits together are called
    _____.

8. A theory concerned with the way in which people explain the causes of their own and
    other people's behaviour is called _____.

9. The inference that an individual's behaviour is caused by something about the person is
    called a(n) _____.

10. The inference that an individual's behaviour is caused by something about the situation
    that the person is in is called a(n) _____.

11. The notion that we make attributions about a person's behaviour by observing the
    things that covary with that behaviour is called the _____.

12. Information about the extent to which other people behave the same way toward the
    same stimulus as the actor does is called _____.

13. Information about the extent to which an actor behaves in the same way toward
    different stimuli is called _____.

14. Information about the extent to which the behaviour of an actor toward a stimulus is the
    same across time and circumstances is called _____.

15. The tendency to overestimate the extent to which people's behaviour is due to internal,
    dispositional factors and to underestimate the role of situational factors is called the
    _____.

16. The tendency to see others' behaviour as dispositionally caused and our own behaviour
    as situationally caused is known as the _____.

17. Explanations for one's successes that credit internal, dispositional factors, and
    explanations for one's failures that blame external, situational factors are called
    _____.

18. A form of defensive attribution wherein people think that good things are more likely to happen to them than to their peers, and that bad things are less likely to happen to them than to their peers is called _____.

19. A form of defensive attribution wherein people assume that bad things happen to bad people and that good things happen to good people is called

_____.

Multiple Choice:

20. Greg has recently taken in a stray dog. If you make an external attribution for Greg's behaviour, you will conclude that:
    a) Greg likes dogs.
    b) Greg felt sorry for the dog.
    c) the dog is probably cute and friendly.
    d) others will perceive Greg as an animal lover.

21. The perception that our own behaviours are caused by the situation but that others' behaviours are dispositionally caused is known as the _____.
    a) fundamental attribution error
    b) attribution difference
    c) actor/observer difference
    d) anchoring adjustment heuristic

22. A consequence of our belief in a just world is that we:
    a) blame the victims of misfortune.
    b) focus on situational causes of others' behaviour.
    c) make accurate attributions and impressions.
    d) are more likely to attribute our own behaviour to dispositional causes.

23. Facial expressions, tone of voice, and the use of touch are all examples of:
    a) context dependent attributional cues.
    b) affect blends.
    c) display rules.
    d) nonverbal communication.

24. Japanese women less often exhibit a wide, uninhibited smile than women in Western cultures because Japanese and Western cultures prescribe different _____.
    a) display rules
    b) values
    c) affect blends
    d) implicit personality theories

25. Which of the following is an example of an emblem?
    a) a road sign
    b) the written explanation of a nonverbal cue
    c) the "okay" sign created with the thumb and forefinger
    d) averted eye gaze

26. The display of different emotions on different parts of the face is called a(n)
    a) affect emblem.
    b) nonverbal blend
    c) facial incongruity
    d) affect blend

27. According to Fritz Heider (1958), the attributions we make for people's behaviour can be either ____ or ____.
    a) target-based; category based
    b) internal; external
    c) perceptual; physical
    d) accurate; biased

28. The three types of information central to Kelly's (1967) covariation model are:
    a) consensus, correspondence, and distinctiveness.
    b) consensus, consistency, and correspondence.
    c) correspondence, distinctiveness, and consistency.
    d) consensus, distinctiveness, and consistency.

29. Research on cultural differences in attributional styles indicates that people from Western cultures are:
    a) less skilled at forming impressions of behaviour.
    b) taught to prefer dispositional explanations of behaviour.
    c) taught to prefer situational explanations of behaviour.
    d) reluctant to publicly state dispositional explanations of behaviour.

30. Research on the accuracy of our first impressions of strangers reveals that:
    a) we are surprisingly accurate in our estimates of people who are similar to us.
    b) we are surprisingly accurate in our estimates of people in general.
    c) we are surprisingly inaccurate when we have little information on which to base our impressions.
    d) our impressions of others become no more accurate the more we get to know them.

31. Though you may have an inaccurate impression of Jane, you may be good at predicting her behaviour when you are together if:
    a) you treat her in such a manner that makes her behaviour confirm your expectancies.
    b) you maintain a high degree of confidence in your predictions.
    c) you make internal attributions for her behaviours.
    d) all of the above

Short Essay

32. Give a recent example of self-serving attributions that you've made for success and failure.

33. Give a recent example of how someone you know was the victim of a crime or illness and was blamed for this outcome.

34.   Give an example of a time you committed the fundamental attribution error. Explain why this might have happened using explanations for the fundamental attribution error from your textbook.

CHAPTER 5

Self-Knowledge: How We Come to Understand Ourselves

CHAPTER OVERVIEW

The first part of Chapter 5 considers the nature of the self and how definitions of the self differ according to culture. The remainder of the chapter documents major theories in social psychology that help us understand how we may find out information about ourselves. Each theory focuses on a different method of discovering self-knowledge. Another difference between the theories presented in the chapter is that some deal with finding out who we are and others deal with finding out how we feel and why. An assumption of these theories is that we do not always know how we feel and why we feel the way we do. Some theories acknowledge that we may be incorrect about our feelings and their origins.

One way to gain self-knowledge is via introspection. Self-awareness theory proposes that by becoming aware of oneself, one can increase self-knowledge. Sometimes self-awareness can be unpleasant, however. A second theory proposes that we gain self-knowledge by examining our own behaviours. The self-perception theory helps us understand how rewards influence our motivation to perform tasks. Two theories in the chapter, the two-factor theory of emotion and the cognitive appraisal theories of emotion, help explain how we experience emotions and how we interpret the causes of our emotions.

Self-schemas are cognitive structures that consist of organised self-knowledge. These schemas assist us in processing new information that may be self-relevant. The importance of autobiographical memories and the possibility of recovering both true and false memories is also discussed in this section. The last section in this chapter focuses on how and why we present ourselves to other people. Our need to engage in impression management is examined as are strategies that allow us to present our desired impressions to others.

CHAPTER OUTLINE

The Nature of the Self

      The Function of the Self

      Cultural Differences in the Definition of the Self

      Gender Differences in the Definition of the Self

Knowing Ourselves through Introspection

      Focusing on the Self: Self-Awareness Theory

      Judging Why We Feel the Way We Do: Telling More than We Can Know

Knowing Ourselves through Observations of Our Own Behaviour

    Inferring Who We Are from How We Behave: Self-Perception Theory

    Intrinsic Motivation versus Extrinsic Motivation

    Understanding Our Emotions: The Two-Factor Theory of Emotion

    Finding the Wrong Cause: Misattribution of Arousal

Knowing Ourselves through Self-Schemas

    Autobiographical Memory

Knowing Ourselves through Social Interaction

    The Looking Glass Self

    Social Comparison Theory

Impression Management: All the World's a Stage

LEARNING OBJECTIVES

After reading Chapter 5, you should be able to do the following:

1.   Define self-concept. Discuss animal and human research on the development of self across species and within humans. Discuss how our self-concepts change with age. (pp. 140-142)

2.   Discuss the three important functions served by the self. (pp. 142-144)

3.   Describe different conceptions of the self across cultures. Contrast the independent view of the self with the interdependent view of the self. (pp. 144-145)

4.   Discuss gender differences in the self-concept in Western Cultures. Discuss the motives that govern how people view themselves. (pp. 145-148)

5.   Discuss introspection as a source of self-knowledge. Describe self-awareness theory and what kinds of information self-awareness reveals. Identify the emotional and behavioural consequences of self-awareness. Discuss when self-awareness is aversive and how we attempt to stop being self-aware. (pp. 148-152)

6.   Distinguish between introspections about how we feel or what kind of person we are, and why we feel the way we do. Discuss the role of causal theories in telling more than we can know.
(pp. 152-154)

7.   Describe the postulates of Daryl Bem's self-perception theory. Identify when and how people use observations of their own behaviour as a source of self-knowledge. (pp. 154-155)

8.   Describe the relationship between intrinsic motivation, external rewards, and the overjustification effect. Define task-contingent and performance-contingent rewards. Identify conditions under which overjustification can be avoided. (pp. 155-160)

9.   Identify the two factors or steps required to understand our own emotional states according to Schachter's two-factor theory of emotion. Discuss the implications of Schachter's theory for the idea that emotions are somewhat arbitrary. Discuss how the two-factor theory explains the misattribution of arousal. (pp. 160-163)

10.   Identify the effects of self-schemas on people's interpretation of new information and on autobiographical memory. (pp. 163-165)

11.   Discuss social interaction as a source of knowledge about ourselves. Define the looking glass self and discuss how it is constructed. (pp. 165-166)

12.   Identify the postulates of social comparison theory. Discuss when people engage in social comparison and with whom they choose to compare themselves when their goal is to construct an accurate self-image. Discuss the motives underlying upward and downward social comparisons and the consequences of engaging in each. (pp. 166-171)

13.   Identify the relationship between self-presentation and impression management. Discuss Goffman's theory of social interaction. (pp. 171-172)

KEY TERMS

self-concept (p. 140)

self-awareness (p. 141)

independent view of the self (p. 144)

interdependent view of the self (p. 144)

introspection (p. 148)

self-awareness theory (p. 149)

causal theories (p. 153)

self-perception theory (p. 155)

intrinsic motivation (p. 155)

extrinsic motivation (p. 155)

overjustification effect (p. 156)

task-contingent rewards (p. 159)

performance-contingent rewards (p. 159)

two-factor theory of emotion (p. 160)

misattribution of arousal (p. 162)

self-schemas (p. 163)

autobiographical memories (p. 164)

looking glass self (p. 165)

social comparison theory (p. 167)

downward social comparison (p. 168)

upward social comparison (p. 169)

self-presentation (p. 171)

impression management (p. 171)

STUDY QUESTIONS

1. What is a self-concept and how does it change from childhood to adulthood?

2. How do self-concepts differ in Western cultures compared to Eastern cultures?

3. How do self-concepts differ according to gender?

4. How often do people rely on introspection for self-knowledge?

5. According to self-awareness theory, what are the consequences of becoming self-aware? What are strategies people use to become less self-aware?

6. When is self-knowledge difficult to obtain? Why do causal theories fall short of explaining why we feel or did something? Why is it a problem to rely on language to describe the origins of our feelings?

7. According to self-perception theory, what besides introspection is a source of self-knowledge? When are we most likely to seek out this source of self-knowledge?

8. What is the overjustification effect? What type of motivation is adversely affected by the overjustification effect? Why is this problematic? Which type of rewards are less likely to result in the overjustification effect?

    — intrinsic motivation
    — performance contingent rewards.

9. According to the two-factor theory of emotion, how do we understand our emotional states? What is the significance of the main findings of the Schachter and Singer (1962) experiment? What is misattribution of arousal?

10. What is a self-schema? What do self-schemas influence? How do self-schemas affect our autobiographical memories?

    — how we interpret new things that happen to us.
    — motivational factor = wanting to see ourselves in a positive light = selective memory;

11. Why is the looking-glass self important for developing a sense of self?

12. Why do we engage in social comparison? What are the consequences of making upward and downward social comparisons? What are motives underlying each type of comparison?

13. How is impression management different from self-presentation? How do we manage our impressions?

PRACTICE QUIZ CHAPTER 5

Fill-in-the-blank

1.   The "known" aspect of the self or the self-definition is called _____.

2.   The process whereby people look inward and examine their own thoughts, feelings, and motives is known as _____.

3.   A theory which states that when people focus their attention on themselves they evaluate and compare their behaviour to their internal standards and values is called _____.

4.   A theory about the causes of one's own feelings and behaviours is called a(n) _____.

5.   One theory maintains that when our attitudes and feelings are uncertain or ambiguous we infer these states by observing our behaviour and the situation in which it occurs. This theory is called _____.

6.   Incentive to engage in an activity because it is enjoyable or interesting is called _____.

7.   The finding that people view their behaviour as caused by compelling extrinsic reasons and underestimate the extent to which their behaviour is caused by intrinsic reasons is termed the _____.

8.   One theory says that people infer what their emotions are by first experiencing physiological arousal and then by using situational cues to suggest an emotional label for that arousal. This theory is called the _____.

9.   Attributing one's arousal to the wrong source, resulting in a mistaken or exaggerated emotion is called _____.

10.   The self we see through the eyes of other people is known as the _____.

11.   A theory which holds that people learn about their own abilities and attitudes by comparing themselves to others is called _____.

12.   Comparing ourselves to people who are better than we are on a particular trait or ability, in order to determine the standard of excellence is called _____.

13.   Providing others with an image of who you are or who you want others to believe you are through your words, nonverbal behaviours, and your actions is called _____.

14. Consciously or unconsciously orchestrating a carefully designed presentation of self that will create a certain impression that fits your goals or needs in social interaction is called _____.

Multiple Choice

15. When asked "Who am I?" a child is most likely to respond
    a) "I'm a nine-year-old."
    b) "I'm a happy person."
    c) "My friends think I'm friendly."
    d) "I'm against corporal punishment."

16. What is most likely an accurate view of the self in people in Eastern cultures?
    a) the independent view
    b) the correspondent view
    c) the interdependent view
    d) the individualistic view

17. Nisbett and Wilson (1977) asked shoppers which pair of identical pantyhose on a display table they preferred and why. Shoppers failed to recognise that the position of the pantyhose caused them to prefer items on the right side of the display because
    a) their causal schemas told them that presenting items on the left causes more favourable evaluations.
    b) participants failed to use causal schemas to make their evaluations.
    c) participants failed to introspect when making their evaluations.
    d) their causal schemas told them that the position of items does not affect preference.

18. According to Daryl Bem's (1972) self-perception theory, when internal cues about attitudes or personality are weak, ambiguous, or uninterpretable, people
    a) cannot form accurate self-perceptions.
    b) engage in introspection to determine how they feel and so clarify the meaning of their internal cues.
    c) compare their behaviours to stronger internal cues such as values and standards for behaviour.
    d) infer their own internal states by observing their own overt behaviour.

19. ____ theory argues that we are rational perceivers trying to form accurate impressions of the world.
    a) Self-perception
    b) Impression management
    c) Attribution
    d) Cognitive Dissonance

20. Giving teenagers extra privileges in exchange for doing household chores will probably not produce the overjustification effect because
    a) extrinsic interest in this activity is initially high.
    b) intrinsic interest in this activity is initially low.
    c) teenagers have already learned to operate within a system of rewards and punishments.
    d) extra privileges are not extrinsic motivators for teenagers.

21. Which type of rewards are more likely to lead to the overjustification effect?
    a) performance-contingent rewards
    b) task-contingent rewards
    c) instrinsic-contingent rewards
    d) response-contingent rewards

22. The two factors in Schachter's (1964) two-factor theory of emotion are
    a) physiological arousal and introspection.
    b) overt behaviour and observing that behaviour from an external perspective.
    c) physiological arousal and seeking a label that explains the arousal.
    d) overt behaviour and seeking an explanation for the behaviour.

23. Which of the following demonstrates the misattribution of arousal?
    a) You rarely pet cats and infer that you do not like them.
    b) You panic in the belief that you will fail an exam after taking two caffeine tablets to get you through an "all-nighter".
    c) You find your job at the bookstore less enjoyable following a substantial raise in pay.
    d) All of the above demonstrate the misattribution of arousal.

24. The looking glass self is constructed as we adopt, over time,
    a) a set of beliefs consistent with our self-concept.
    b) the ability to compare ourselves to others.
    c) the ability to manage the self we present to others.
    d) other people's perspectives of us.

25. Which of the following theories begins with the supposition that people have a need to evaluate their opinions and abilities?
    a) impression management theory
    b) the two factor theory of emotion
    c) social comparison theory
    d) self-perception theory

26. Which of the following is true about introspection?
    a) Males are more introspective than females.
    b) Introspection is useful in explaining why we feel or behave the way we do.
    c) As an internal process, it cannot be initiated by external factors.
    d) We do not rely on this source of information as often as we think we do.

27. Deciding that you are in a bad mood because it is Monday is an example of a(n)
   a)   availability heuristic.
   b)   causal theory.
   c)   perceptual set.
   d)   self-schema.

28. Which of the following demonstrates the overjustification effect?
   a)   A band member enjoys her job as a guitarist in a band and decides to go solo.
   b)   Hugo loves to read and joins a book club that requires a monthly fee.
   c)   Pamela quits her job as a secretary because she finds it boring and goes back to school.
   d)   An engineer who loved to solve mechanical problems as a child now views them as dreary tasks.

29. Participants in a study by Schachter and Singer (1962) who unwittingly took epinephrine, a drug that causes arousal, felt angry when filling out an insulting questionnaire in the presence of another angry individual because
   a)   epinephrine made them angry.
   b)   they experienced arousal and sought out an explanation or label for that arousal in the situation.
   c)   the epinephrine heightened the feeling of annoyance produced by the questionnaire.
   d)   heightened arousal enabled subjects to experience empathy for the other individual and so experience his anger.

30. Organised knowledge structures about ourselves, based on our past experiences, that help us understand, explain, and predict our own behaviour are known as
   a)   introspective schemas.
   b)   internal attributions.
   c)   self-schemas.
   d)   autobiographical memories.

31. Ross (1989) found that when it comes to their attitudes regarding important social issues, people tend to
   a)   overestimate how stable their attitudes are.
   b)   accurately perceive that their attitudes change with changes in social norms.
   c)   accurately perceive that these attitudes are highly stable.
   d)   underestimate how stable their attitudes are.

32. In order to gain important self-knowledge, people choose to compare themselves to
   a)   others who are similar to them on the important attribute or dimension.
   b)   individuals regarded as "typical" on the important attribute or dimension.
   c)   individuals regarded as "the best" on the important attribute or dimension.
   d)   others who are inferior to them on the important attribute or dimension.

Short Essay

33. Argue that self-perception theory is a variation on attribution theory discussed in Chapter 4.

34. You have been dating someone for a week now and have decided that before the relationship goes any further that it would be a good idea to introspect about the reasons WHY you like this person. What is likely to happen as you introspect? What negative consequence might arise from your introspection?

35. What are the advantages and disadvantages of self-awareness?

36. Compare and contrast self-perception theory and the two-factor theory of emotion.

37. You have worked in the library for two years. One year ago, if someone had asked you how much you liked your job, you would have said that you liked it very much. Since then, you have received a large raise in pay. Why, if you overjustify your reason for working at the library, will you claim to like the job less following your raise?

38. What is the looking glass self and how is it constructed? What research suggests that social interaction is necessary for the development of the self?

CHAPTER 6

Self-Justification and the Need to Maintain Self-Esteem

CHAPTER OVERVIEW

Chapter 6 focuses on the consequences of the need we have to justify our actions in order to maintain our self-esteem. The first part of the chapter discusses the need to feel good about ourselves. The focus of self-discrepancy theory is how inconsistencies within aspects of one's self create distress. Self-completion theory explains how when an aspect of the self-concept is threatened, social recognition for that aspect of the self-concept is sought. Self-evaluative maintenance theory proposes that the self-concept can be threatened by the behaviour of someone close to us if that behaviour is personally relevant to us. Self-affirmation theory suggests that threats to the self-concept are addressed by reflecting on areas of competence different from the threat. The second part of the chapter looks at self-evaluation. Sometimes we want to feel good about ourselves regardless of the truth, but sometimes we desire confirmation of our self-concept that is accurate.

The final part of the chapter examines cognitive dissonance theory. Cognitive dissonance theory assists us in making sense of people's feelings and behaviours that may seem counter-intuitive. Making irrevocable decisions, expending effort to attain a goal, and counterattitudinal advocacy can all result in dissonance. Since dissonance is perceived as unpleasant, different ways to reduce dissonance exist and are described.

CHAPTER OUTLINE

The Need to Feel Good about Ourselves

       Self-Discrepancy Theory

       Self-Completion Theory

       Self-Evaluation Maintenance Theory

       Self-Affirmation Theory

Self-Evaluation: Biased or Accurate?

       Self-Enhancement: Wanting to Feel Good about Ourselves, Regardless of the Facts

       Self-Verification: Wanting to Know the Truth about Ourselves

The Need to Justify Our Actions

       The Theory of Cognitive Dissonance

       Decisions, Decisions, Decisions

       The Justification of Effort

The Psychology of Insufficient Justification

The Evidence for Motivational Arousal

The Aftermath of Good and Bad Deeds

Avoiding the Rationalization Trap

Learning from Our Mistakes

The Solar Temple Revisited

LEARNING OBJECTIVES

After reading Chapter 6, you should be able to do the following:

1.   Define self-discrepancy theory. Discuss consequences of conflict between the actual self and the ideal self and ought selves. Describe how distress due to self-discrepancy can be reduced. (pp. 178-179)

2.   Define self-completion theory. Describe how a positive self-image can be maintained according to this theory. (pp. 179-180)

3.   Describe self-evaluation maintenance theory and the conditions when we bask in the reflected glory of a friend's achievements. Describe the methods used to deal with threats to our self-esteem. (pp. 180-184)

4.   Define self-affirmation theory. Describe the conditions under which self-affirmation will be used to reduce dissonance. Describe the relationship between self-affirmation and culture. (pp. 184-187)

5.   Define self-enhancement and self-verification theories and compare the two theories. (pp. 187-192)

6.   Describe the theory of cognitive dissonance. Discuss the conditions that elicit dissonance and what strategies we use to reduce dissonance. (pp. 192-194)

7.   Define post-decision dissonance. Explain how changing our attitudes after a decision serves to reduce dissonance. (pp. 195-198)

8.   Define what is meant by justification of effort. Identify the consequences of working hard to attain something and the importance of volunteering such effort. (pp. 198-201)

9.   Distinguish between internal and external justification. Define counter-attitudinal advocacy. Describe the effects of inducing counter-attitudinal advocacy with minimum external justification. Describe how dissonance theory has been applied to AIDS prevention. (pp. 201-204)

10. Explain how insufficient punishment leads to self-persuasion. Describe the effects of self-persuasion on behaviour. (pp. 204-206)

11. Discuss evidence for a motivational component to dissonance. (pp. 206-208)

12. Discuss the effects of doing favours for people we do not like and the effects of harming others. Identify the causes and consequences of dehumanising victims. (pp. 208-211)

13. Define a "rationalization trap." How can we avoid it? Describe the relationship between self-affirmation and the rationalization trap. (pp. 211-214)

KEY TERMS

self-discrepancy theory (p. 178)

self-completion theory (p. 179)

self-evaluation maintenance theory (p. 181)

self-affirmation theory (p. 184)

self-enhancement (p. 187)

self-verification theory (p. 190)

cognitive dissonance (p. 192)

postdecision dissonance (p. 195)

justification of effort (p. 199)

external justification (p. 201)

internal justification (p. 201)

counter-attitudinal advocacy (p. 201)

insufficient punishment (p. 204)

self-justification (p. 205)

rationalization trap (p. 211)

STUDY QUESTIONS

1. What does self-discrepancy theory explain? How do we cope with the negative feelings generated by self-discrepancy according to this theory?

   - that we become distressed when our sense of who we truly are (actu. self) is discrepant from our personal std or desired self-conceptions.
   - Try to interpret performance in most positive light poss (self protective stratagy)
     → shud reasses situation, expend more effort.

2. What is self-completion theory? How are threats to the self concept addressed according to this theory?

   - when people exp. a threat to a valued aspect of self-concept, they become highly motivated to seek social recognition of that identity.
   - look for ways to signal to others that we have a credible, legit. claim to a partic. identity.

3. What is self-evaluation maintenance theory? What determines the perceived level of threat according to this theory? How does this theory explain why people may help strangers more than they help their friends?

   - theory that one's self concept can be threatened by another's behaviour — level of threat determined by closeness to person & relevance of the behaviour.
   - out performance by friends threatens self-esteem.

4. How does self-affirmation affect dissonance-arousing threat?

   - reduces dissonance-arousing threat to self-concept by focusing on & affirming competence on some dimension unrelated to the threat.

5. What are conditions that may result in cognitive dissonance? Why does cognitive dissonance occur?

   - feeling of discomfort caused by inconsistency between behaviour / attitudes or 2 conflicting attitudes.
   - motivates person to reduce discomfort: 1) changing behaviour
                                            2) changing cognitions
                                            3) adding new cognitions

6. What is the relationship between making important decisions and experiencing dissonance? What happens to attitudes toward the chosen alternative and the unchosen alternative? How does the permanence of the decision affect the experience of dissonance?

7. How does dissonance reduction after a moral decision affect people's tendency to behave ethically or unethically in the future?

8. What is the relationship between the justification of effort and dissonance reduction?

52

9.   Why can insufficient justification result in dissonance? What are the consequences of reducing dissonance through external justification compared to internal justification? When does counterattitudinal advocacy result in private attitude change?

→ w/a minimum of external justification.

10.   What are the effects of insufficient punishment on the judgements of an object or entity? What are the effects of mild versus severe threats on the level of dissonance experienced?

11.   What are the consequences of doing something unpleasant for a friend compared to doing something unpleasant for someone who is disliked? What are the effects of doing a favour for someone on how much this person is liked? How and why does dehumanising victims occur?

12.   What is a rationalization trap and how does one develop? How can this trap be avoided?

PRACTICE QUIZ CHAPTER 6

Fill-in-the-blank

1.   A feeling of discomfort caused by performing an action that is discrepant from one's conception of oneself as a decent and sensible person is called
_____.

2.   Dissonance that is aroused after a person makes a decision is called
_____.

3.   The tendency for people to increase their liking for something they have worked hard to attain is called _____.

4.   A person's reason or explanation for his/her dissonant behaviour that resides outside the individual is known as _____.

5.   Reducing dissonance by changing something about oneself is called
_____.

6.   A process by which individuals are induced to state an opinion or attitude that runs counter to their own private belief or attitude is called a
_____.

7. External justification that is insufficient for having resisted a desired activity or object and which usually results in individuals devaluing the activity or object is called _____.

8. A theory suggesting that people will reduce the impact of a dissonance arousing threat by focusing on and affirming their competence on some dimension unrelated to the threat is called _____.

9. A theory suggesting that people have a need to seek confirmation of their self-concept, whether the self-concept is positive or negative, is called _____.

10. The web of distortion that we trap ourselves in by rationalising past behaviours and that prevents us from seeing things as they really are is called the _____.

11. The tendency to justify one's actions in order to maintain one's self-esteem is called _____.

12. _____ theory states that we become upset when our actual self is different form our personal standards.

13. A statement that is contrary to private beliefs or attitudes is called _____.

Multiple Choice

14. An individual who strongly opposes helmet laws is excited to find a study which shows that neck injuries are a more common outcome of motorcycle accidents when helmets are worn than when helmets are not worn. This individual is reducing dissonance by
    a) changing behaviour to bring it in line with the dissonant cognition.
    b) adding cognitions that justify the behaviour.
    c) modifying dissonant cognitions to justify the behaviour.
    d) adopting a self-concept that is consistent with the behaviour.

15. If a participant in Brehm's (1956) study claimed that an iron and an electric can opener were equally desirable appliances, she was asked to choose one of these as a gift. Later she was asked to re-rate the two appliances. If she chose the can opener, her second rating of the appliances were typically
    a) lower for the can opener and higher for the iron.
    b) lower for the can opener and lower for the iron.
    c) higher for the can opener and higher for the iron.
    d) higher for the can opener and lower for the iron.

16. Mills (1958) had children compete on a difficult exam under conditions that made cheating easy and presumably undetectable. The children's attitudes toward cheating were measured the next day and revealed that
   a) children who cheated adopted a harsher attitude toward cheating while those who resisted cheating became more lenient toward cheating.
   b) children adopted a more lenient attitude toward cheating after competing with each other.
   c) children who cheated became more lenient toward cheating while those who resisted cheating adopted a harsher attitude toward cheating.
   d) children became more lenient toward cheating after competing with each other.

17. In the Festinger and Carlsmith (1959) experiment, participants who were paid $20.00 to lie felt less dissonance than subjects paid $1.00 because receiving $20.00
   a) put participants in a good mood that counteracted dissonance.
   b) provided self-verification cues that participants were in fact moral people.
   c) was sufficient external justification for lying.
   d) allowed subjects to affirm their worth and circumvented dissonance.

18. Dehumanising the victim increases
   a) dissonance caused by our cruel treatment of others.
   b) the likelihood that cruel treatment will continue or even escalate.
   c) empathy for the victim.
   d) the likelihood that hostilities will end.

19. According to self-evaluation maintenance theory, we want our friends to do well on tasks of low self-relevance so that we can
   a) bask in the reflected glory of our friends' achievements.
   b) distract our friends from excelling on tasks of high self-relevance.
   c) make the task more relevant to ourselves.
   d) provide some distance between ourselves and our friends.

20. Which of the following best characterises the role of self-enhancement needs in people with poor opinions of themselves?
   a) People with poor opinions of themselves are not motivated by self-enhancement needs.
   b) People with poor opinions of themselves feel an especially great need for self-enhancement.
   c) Among people with poor opinions of themselves, the need for self-enhancement is likely to conflict with self-verification needs.
   d) Among people with poor opinions of themselves, self-enhancement is likely to be self-verifying.

21. In order to learn from our mistakes, we must be able to
   a) circumvent dissonance by affirming our positive qualities.
   b) find both internal and external justification for our behaviours.
   c) deny the existence of inconsistent beliefs.
   d) tolerate dissonance long enough to examine the situation objectively.

22. In general, the most rational way to reduce dissonance that follows foolish or immoral behaviour is to
    a) justify the behaviour by adding cognitions to support it.
    b) justify the behaviour by modifying dissonant cognitions.
    c) change the behaviour to bring it in line with the dissonant cognition.
    d) adopt a self-concept that is consistent with the behaviour.

23. Imagine that you've agreed to buy a notoriously unreliable but attractive sports car in favour of a less attractive but dependable station wagon. Which of the following will reduce dissonance in this situation?
    a) knowing that you've purchased an unreliable car
    b) thinking that you could rely on the station wagon
    c) putting a substantial down payment on the sports car
    d) imagining how good you'll look in the sports car

24. When a counter-attitudinal advocacy is accomplished with a minimum of external justification,
    a) private attitudes change in the direction of public statements.
    b) public statements change in the direction of private attitudes.
    c) private attitudes and public statements tend to spread apart.
    d) private attitudes are subtly revealed in public statements.

25. Aronson and Carlsmith (1963) told children that they were not allowed to play with a highly desirable toy and measured the children's liking for the toy after this rule was obeyed in the experimenter's absence. They found that children's liking for the toy
    a) increased when the rule was accompanied by a mild threat.
    b) decreased when the rule was accompanied by a severe threat.
    c) decreased when the rule was accompanied by a mild threat.
    d) increased when the experimenter left the room.

26. Dissonance theory predicts that if we do a favour for someone we dislike, we will
    a) expect a favour in return.
    b) come to like that person.
    c) feel that we are weak.
    d) expect to be taken advantage of.

27. Zanna and Cooper (1974) had participants write a dissonance-producing counter-attitudinal essay after ingesting a placebo that would supposedly arouse or relax them. The greatest attitude change occurred when participants believed that the arousal they felt was being
    a) caused by the placebo.
    b) masked by the placebo.
    c) enhanced by the placebo.
    d) caused by writing the essay.

28. If we cannot rationalise away a threat to our self-esteem we can avoid dissonance by asserting our competence and integrity in some other area. This is the rationale of _____ theory.
   a) self-affirmation
   b) self-evaluation maintenance
   c) self-verification
   d) cognitive dissonance

29. Through the reduction of dissonance, there is a tendency to catch ourselves up in a web of distortion that prevents us from seeing things as they really are. This phenomenon is known as the _____.
   a) distortion web
   b) rationalization trap
   c) ego-defensive snare
   d) self-verification lure

Short Essay

30. How do groups ensure the loyalty of their members by requiring them to endure severe initiation procedures before joining?

31. Contrast the experience of threat described in self-completion theory compared to self-discrepancy theory.

32. The D.J. on the radio congratulates caller number ten. She's just won a prize and is asked what her favourite radio station is. Ecstatically, she replies "W...", the station's call letters. Why is her subsequent opinion of the station likely to be higher if her prize was a T-shirt than if her prize was $100?

33. Experimental participants who voluntarily wrote a counter-attitudinal essay showed the most attitude change when they had taken a placebo that was supposed to relax them. How does this finding support the existence of physiological arousal in dissonance?

CHAPTER 7

Attitudes and Attitude Change: Influencing Thoughts and Feelings

CHAPTER OVERVIEW

In Chapter 7, the topics of attitudes and attitude change are examined. You will discover where attitudes come from in terms of affectively based, behaviourally based or cognitively based. Determinants of attitude strength such as ambivalence, accessibility, subjective experience and autobiographical recall are all discussed.

Attitudes are also studied for their predictive value. Conditions that increase the consistency between attitudes and spontaneous and deliberative behaviours are reviewed.

Attitude change models are discussed in the next section. The precursors and consequences of two routes to persuasion, the central and the peripheral, are addressed. The chapter discusses why and how advertising is effective at changing the buying behaviour of consumers. The controversial topic of subliminal advertising is also presented. Lastly, the chapter provides information on how to resist attitude change through attitude inoculation procedures.

CHAPTER OUTLINE

The Nature and Origin of Attitudes

      Where Do Attitudes Come From?

      Determinants of Attitude Strength

When Will Attitudes Predict Behaviour?

      Predicting Spontaneous Behaviours

      Predicting Deliberate Behaviours

      Attitude-Behaviour Consistency: Implications for Safe Sex

Attitude Change

      Persuasive Communications and Attitude Change

      Fear and Attitude Change

      Advertising and Attitude Change

How to Make People Resistant to Attitude Change

    Attitude Innoculation

    Resisting Peer Pressure

    When Persuasion Attempts Boomerang: Reactance Theory

LEARNING OBJECTIVES

After reading Chapter 7, you should be able to do the following:

1.   Define an attitude and identify its components. Discuss the differences between cognitively based, affectively based and behaviourally based attitudes. Explain how affectively based attitudes are formed via classical conditioning and instrumental conditioning. (pp. 220-225)

2.   Identify different determinants of attitude strength. Discuss the relationship between attitude strength and an attitude's ambivalence, accessibility, subjective experience, and autobiographical recall. (pp. 225-228)

3.   Describe the circumstances when attitudes predict behaviour? Differentiate between predicting spontaneous behaviours versus predicting deliberative behaviours. Discuss the theory of planned behaviour as an explanation for predicting deliberative behaviours. (pp. 228-233)

4.   Discuss the implications of attitude-behaviour consistency for safe sex practices. (pp. 233-235)

5.   Describe the Yale Attitude Change Approach. Identify and define the three factors in an influence setting emphasized by this approach. Provide examples of each factor. Identify a problem with the Yale Attitude Change Approach. (pp. 235-238)

6.   Describe the aim of attitude change models like Petty and Cacioppo's Elaboration Likelihood Model and Chaiken's Systematic-Heuristic Persuasion Model. (pp. 238-239)

7.   Identify factors that increase people's motivation and ability to pay attention to the arguments. Discuss how attitudes changed by the central route to persuasion differ from attitudes changed by the peripheral route. Define need for cognition and discuss its role in persuasion.
(pp. 240-243)

8.   Identify the role of emotional influences and fear-arousing communications in persuasion. Describe the conditions under which fear appeals foster or inhibit attitude change via the central route. (pp. 244-246)

9.   Discuss applications of attitude change to persuasion. What does the research say about negative advertising? (pp. 247-250)

10. Discuss the effectiveness of subliminal advertising. (pp. 250-253)

11. Identify the purpose of attitude inoculation. Identify a potential disadvantage of making people resistant to attitude change. Discuss the role of reactance when persuasion attempts "boomerang". Discuss resisting peer influence. (pp. 253-256)

KEY TERMS

attitude (p. 220)

cognitively based attitude (p. 221)

affectively based attitude (p. 221)

classical conditioning (p. 222)

operant conditioning (p. 222)

behaviourally based attitude (p. 223)

attitude accessibility (p. 226)

theory of planned behaviour (p. 230)

subjective norms (p. 231)

persuasive communication (p. 236)

Yale Attitude Change approach (p. 237)

heuristic-systematic model of persuasion (p. 238)

elaboration likelihood model (p. 238)

need for cognition (p. 241)

fear-arousing communication (p. 246)

subliminal messages (p. 250)

attitude inoculation (p. 253)

reactance theory (p. 256)

STUDY QUESTIONS

1. What is an attitude and what are its components? Why is it important to consider each of these components?
    - an enduring evaluation of a person, object, or idea.
    - components = cognitively-based attitude = based primarily on beliefs about object
        = affectively-based   "   =   "   "   on feelings & values of object
        = behaviourally-based   "   =   "   "   on observations of actions toward
                                                                an object
                                                            - attitudes not based proportion
                                                            diff attitudes have diff. ba
                                                            (eg. reg. groups = cogn based
                                                                pos. "   = affective base

2. What are the origins and aspects of affectively based attitudes?
    - stem from people's values; sensory reaction (eg. chocolate);
    classical cond: neutral stimulus exp. w/an emotional
    response takes on emotional properties (eg. mothballs; grandma);
    operant cond: behaviour increase/decrease w/pos. reinforcement or
                                                        reinforcement (eg. racist attitudes).

3. When do people infer their attitudes from their behaviour?
    - when attitudes weak or ambiguous &
    - when no other plausible explanations for behaviour

4. What is the relationship between attitude accessibility and attitude strength? How does an attitude become accessible?
    - accessibility = 1 of 4 major determinants of attitude strength (others are
    ambivalence, subj. experience; autobiographical recall).
    - expressing an attitude increases its accessibility — (expressing the opposite attitude
    does too).   * The more accessible = stronger; harder to change.

5. When does counterattitudinal advocacy lead to private attitude change? What is the process underlying this change?
    - when reminds us of our true attitude; thereby strengthens the
    accessibility of the attitude ⇒ stronger; less likely to change.

6. According to the Yale Attitude Change Approach, what are the three main elements in a persuasive situation?
    - source of comm. or who is the speaker
    - nature of   "   or   what ⇒ nature of comm. (one-sided vs. 2-sided arguments)
    - nature of audience or who ⇒ age, distraction; intelligence.

7. What are the major differences between the central and peripheral routes to persuasion? What are people attending to when they use each route? When are people more likely to use the central route compared to the peripheral route? What are two motives for the use of the central route, according to the elaboration likelihood model?
    - central = (systematic processing) = pay attn to facts/logic; carefully process ⇒ when pay attn.
                                                                                        motivated to
    - peripheral = (heuristic processing) = mental shortcuts, surface characteristics of message ⇒ when
    not motivated to pay attn.
    ⇒ 2 motives = motivation & ability to pay attn. (if interested & not distracted).

8. What are some examples of peripheral cues? What route to persuasion leads to lasting attitude change?
    - length of comm., attributes of communicator (eg. expert, attractive).
    - central route = enduring, resistant attitudes.

9. How do emotions, like moods, influence persuasion? How do emotions act as a heuristic to persuasion and what route to persuasion are people taking when they use their emotions as a guide to attitude formation?

- good moods = peripheral route b/c avoid activities that may ruin mood.
- sad/neutral moods = central route, analyze comm. in detail.

10. What level of fear is most effective in a persuasive communication? What is the best strategy if you are hoping to arouse fear in your persuasive communication? Why?

- moderate fear w/ humour : specific recommendations for performing desired behaviours.

11. What are important factors to consider when designing a persuasive communication?

- whether interested in creating long-lasting attitude change (central vs. peripheral)
- tailoring to people's attitudes; negative advertising, cultural diffs, subliminal?

12. What is the purpose of attitude inoculation and how should this process be implemented? What is reactance and how may it occur?

- process of making people immune to attempts to change their attitudes by exposing them to small doses of arguments against their position (gives opportunity to think about)
- when people feel threatened, freedom unpleasant state is reduced by reactance — performing the threatened behaviour.

13. Under what conditions do attitudes predict spontaneous and deliberative behaviours? How does the theory of planned behaviour predict deliberative behaviours?

- attitudes predict spontaneous behaviour only when highly accessible (eg. snap decisions).
- deliberate behaviours follow the Theory of Planned Behaviour : depends on 1) attitudes towards specific behaviour (not general attitude) eg. birth control pills during next 2 years 2) their subjective norms - beliefs re: how others care about a behaviour 3) perceived behavioural control

14. Is there evidence that subliminal messages in a persuasive communication influence our behaviour in everyday life?

eg. if believe easy, will set strong intention to perform.

- no; ineffective in everyday life, although evidence in lab studies.
- ads are more powerful when we consciously perceive them.

15. How do ads perpetuate stereotypical patterns of thinking? Provide examples.

PRACTICE QUIZ CHAPTER 7

Fill-in-the-Blank

1. An enduring evaluation--positive or negative--of people, objects, and ideas is called a(n) _____.

2. The component of an attitude comprised of the emotions and feelings people associate with an attitude object is called the _____ component.

3. The component of an attitude comprised of people's beliefs about the properties of the attitude object is called the _____ component.

4. The component of an attitude comprised of people's actions toward the attitude object is called the _____ component.

5. The study of the conditions under which people are most likely to change their attitudes in response to persuasive messages is called the _____.

6. A theory which specifies when people will take the central or peripheral route to persuasion when presented with a persuasive communication is called the _____.

7. The route to persuasion people take when they carefully think about and process the content of a persuasive communication is called the _____ route.

8. The route to persuasion people take when they are persuaded by surface characteristics of a persuasive communication is called the _____ route.

9. Persuasive messages that attempt to change people's attitudes by arousing their fears are called _____.

10. Attitudes that are based primarily on people's beliefs about the properties of the attitude object are called _____.

11. Attitudes that are based primarily on people's emotions and values that are evoked by the attitude object are called _____.

12. The process of repeatedly pairing an emotion-evoking stimulus with a neutral stimulus until the neutral stimulus takes on the emotional properties of the first stimulus is called _____.

13. Changing the frequency of freely chosen behaviours by positively reinforcing or punishing the behaviour is called _____.

14. Attitudes that are based primarily on people's observations of how they behave toward the attitude object are called _____.

15. The strength of association between an object and a person's evaluation of that object is known as _____.

16. Making people immune to attitude change attempts by initially exposing them to small doses of the arguments against their position is called _____.

17. According to one theory, when people feel that their freedom to perform a certain behaviour is threatened, they will reduce the threat by performing that behaviour. This theory is called _____.

18. According to one theory, the best predictors of people's planned, deliberative behaviours are people's attitudes toward the specific behaviour, their subjective norms, and their perceived behavioural control. This theory is called the
_____.

19. People's beliefs about how other people they care about will view their behaviour are called their _____.

20. Words and pictures which are not consciously perceived but supposedly influential are called _____.

Multiple Choice

21. Responding to a "puppies for sale" ad, you arrive at the seller's home and immediately fall in love with the first puppy you see. The component of your attitude toward the puppy which is exemplified by such a reaction is called the ____ component.
   a)   behavioural
   b)   cognitive
   c)   affective
   d)   heuristic

22. While studying the conditions under which people are most likely to be influenced by persuasive communications, Hovland and colleagues at Yale repeatedly asked
   a)   who says what to whom?
   b)   when will logical arguments persuade people and when will more superficial characteristics do so?
   c)   why are communications persuasive?
   d)   what condition produces the most influence?

23. Distraction during a persuasive message and message complexity prevent the careful consideration of relevant arguments by decreasing the
   a)   motivation to attend to relevant arguments.
   b)   ability to attend to relevant arguments.
   c)   personal relevance of the message.
   d)   degree of association between message characteristics and internal response cues.

24. Though fear-arousing communications are threatening, people will reduce this threat by changing their attitudes and behaviours only when
   a)   the communication produces an extremely high level of fear.
   b)   the fear-arousing message can be easily ignored.
   c)   the fear-arousing communication is directed at individuals with high levels of self-esteem.
   d)   the fear-arousing communication offers suggestions about how to avoid the threat.

25. Children may adopt prejudiced attitudes through operant conditioning if their parents
    a) associate such attitudes with emotionally positive stimuli.
    b) punish them for expressing such attitudes.
    c) reward them for expressing such attitudes.
    d) present arguments favouring such attitudes.

26. A personality variable that has been linked to the use of the central route to persuasion is:
    a) need for emotion
    b) need for reason
    c) need for explanation
    d) need for cognition

27. Good moods are most likely to result in taking the ____ route to persuasion.
    a) central
    b) heuristic
    c) peripheral
    d) cognitive

28. Words or pictures that are not consciously perceived but may be influential are:
    a) exceptional messages
    b) subliminal messages
    c) reactance messages
    d) unconscious messages

29. The theory of planned behaviour states that all of the following are predictors of people's planned, deliberative behaviours EXCEPT
    a) subjective norms
    b) perceived behavioural control
    c) attitudes toward the specific behaviour
    d) social norms

30. According to Petty and Cacioppo's (1986) Elaboration Likelihood Model, when people are persuaded by surface characteristics of a message, such as how long the message is, they have taken the ____ route to persuasion.
    a) central
    b) peripheral
    c) heuristic
    d) subjective

31. Attitudes changed by the central route to persuasion are
    a) maintained over time.
    b) consistent with behaviours.
    c) resistant to counterpersuasion.
    d) all of the above

32. When you encounter an object and your attitude toward that object comes immediately to mind, your attitude is said to be highly ____.
   a)   resistant
   b)   accessible
   c)   deliberative
   d)   intentional

33. After strongly prohibiting the reading of banned books, professor Jones has noticed an increased interest by her students in the books. Which of the following theories best explains this outcome?
   a)   theory of reasoned action
   b)   elaboration likelihood model
   c)   reactance theory
   d)   classical conditioning theory

34. Responses to which of the following questions will best predict whether someone donates clothes to the Salvation Army next Sunday at noon?
   a)   "How much are you willing to help others"?
   b)   "How do you feel about making donations to charities"?
   c)   "How do you feel about donating clothes to the Salvation Army"?
   d)   "How do you feel about donating clothes to the Salvation Army next Sunday at noon"?

Short Essay

35. Give examples of cognitively, affectively, and behaviourally based attitudes.

36. When do persuasive attempts "boomerang" and why?

37. As a marketing specialist, what advertising approach would you recommend to the maker of greeting cards?

38. Describe Petty and Cacioppo's (1986) Elaboration Likelihood Model. What are the two routes to persuasion that people may take? What determines the route taken? What are the effects of persuasion by each route?

39. Describe the "attitude inoculation" technique used to help people resist attempts to persuade them. How has this technique been adapted in order to make individuals resistant to peer pressure?

CHAPTER 8

Conformity: Influencing Behaviour

CHAPTER OVERVIEW

This chapter deals with the powerful influence that others have to get us to do what they are doing or what they want us to do. The first section of the chapter describes one type of influence that increases conformity, informational social influence. The motivation to be right underlies informational social influence. Although it is adaptive to follow others when they are right, the chapter warns us that resisting informational social influence may be best sometimes. Steps to do this are outlined.

Another type of influence linked with conformity is normative social influence. Classic studies are depicted in this section that made us aware of our concern to adhere to social norms and be liked by others. This is the motivation that underlies normative social influence. As with informational social influence, resisting normative pressures is possible. Another topic addressed in this section is minority influence. Minority influence research studies how small groups can influence larger ones.

The next section of this chapter considers compliance. Compliance involves changing one's behaviour as a result of a direct request from someone. A particular kind of conformity, obedience to authority, is addressed. The findings of Milgram comprise the bulk of this material. His studies of obedience have contributed greatly to our understanding of how people can commit inhumane acts by virtue of situational constraints.

CHAPTER OUTLINE

Conformity: When and Why

Informational Social Influence: The Need To Know What's "Right"

      When Will People Conform to Informational Social Influence?

      When Informational Conformity Backfires

      Resisting Informational Social Influence

Normative Social Influence: The Need to Be Accepted

      Conformity and Social Approval: The Asch Line Judgement Studies

      When Will People Conform to Normative Social Influence?

      Resisting Normative Social Influence

Social Influence in Everyday Life

Minority Influence: When the Few Influence the Many

Compliance: Requests to Change Your Behaviour

       The Door-in-the-Face Technique

       The Foot-in-the-Door Technique

       Lowballing

Obedience to Authority

       The Role of Normative Social Influence

       The Role of Informational Social Influence

       Other Reasons Why We Obey

LEARNING OBJECTIVES

After reading Chapter 8, you should be able to do the following:

1.   Define conformity and give some examples. (pp. 261-262)

2.   Identify the motivation underlying informational social influence. Describe Sherif's (1936) experiment. (pp. 262-263)

3.   Distinguish between private acceptance and public compliance. (p. 264)

4.   Identify the conditions under which informational social influence produces conformity. (pp. 264-268)

5.   Identify the steps people can take to determine whether other people provide accurate information and to resist other people's information when it is inaccurate. (pp. 268-270)

6.   Identify the motivation underlying normative social influence. Define and give examples of social norms. (pp. 270-271)

7.   Describe Asch's (1956) experiment. Identify how the situation in Asch's experiment differed from the situation in Sherif's experiment. Describe the basic findings of Asch's experiment. Explain why these findings were surprising. (pp. 271-274)

8.   Identify when people will conform to normative social influence. Describe social impact theory. Describe the predictions made by social impact theory based on group size, importance, unanimity, possessing people of a certain type, and collectivist. (pp. 274-280)

9.   Discuss the consequences of resisting normative social influence. Describe Schachter's (1951) experiment and discuss its results. (pp. 280-282)

10. Discuss examples of normative social influence from harmless trends and fads to forms of conformity including many women's and men's attempts to conform to a body image dictated by society. (pp. 282-286)

11. Discuss the necessity of minority influence for introducing change in groups. Identify how a minority must express its views if it is to exert influence. Identify the kind of social influence minorities exert and what effect this has on the majority. (pp. 286-287)

12. Define compliance. Discuss the relationship between the door-in-the-face technique and the reciprocity norm. Identify a disadvantage of the door-in-the-face technique. (pp. 287-289)

13. Define the foot-in-the-door technique and lowballing. (pp. 289-291)

14. Describe Milgram's obedience studies. Discuss variations of the original study which demonstrate the kinds of social influence that caused obedience. Identify key aspects of the situation that caused participants in Milgram's obedience studies to continue following an "obey authority" norm long after it was appropriate to do so. Discuss the roles of normative and informational influence in explaining Milgram's findings. (pp. 291-298)

15. Discuss other reasons we conform. (pp. 298-300)

KEY TERMS

conformity (p. 261)

informational social influence (p. 262)

private acceptance (p. 264)

public compliance (p. 264)

contagion (p. 265)

normative social influence (p. 270)

social norms (p. 270)

social impact theory (p. 274)

idiosyncrasy credits (p. 282)

minority influence (p. 286)

compliance (p. 287)

door-in-the-face technique (p. 287)

reciprocity norm (p. 288)

foot-in-the-door technique (p. 289)

lowballing (p. 290)

obedience (p. 292)

STUDY QUESTIONS

1. What are two main reasons why we conform? What advantages does conforming provide? 1) The need to know what's right ⇒ appropriate behaviour 2) The need to be accepted ⇒ rather than rejection & ridicule.

    - helps us choose appropriate behaviour in ambiguous situations & crises, & social approval.

2. When are we likely to conform to informational social influence? Contrast private acceptance with public compliance. Which one is more likely when we conform due to informational social influence?

    - when a situation is ambiguous; when the situation is a crisis; when an expert is present.
    - private = genuine belief of appropriateness of others' behaviour; public = conforming w/o believing appropriateness of behaviour. — private acceptance more likely w/ informational social infl.

3. Why are times of crises related to an increase in conformity due to informational social influence? What is contagion?

    - usually b/c no time to think & reflect on actions, fear & panic.
    - contagion = rapid transmission of emotions or behaviour thru a crowd.

    (however, can be irrational).

4. What are three main factors that make conforming due to informational social influence very likely? Explain.

    1) when sit = ambiguous → look to others for correct response
    2) when sit = crisis → w/ uncertainty, fear, panic, look to others for correct response
    3) when expert present → w/ knowledge, this person becomes valuable as a guide in above situations.

5. Why is the decision of whether or not to conform so important? What are some questions we should ask ourselves when we are deciding whether we should conform due to informational social influence? - influences how people define reality.
    - if others are misinformed, will lead to inappropriate/inaccurate behaviour.
    → remember it is poss. to resist illegitimate/inaccurate informational social infl.
       1) Do others know more than you? 3) Is others' actions sensible?
       2) Is there an expert who knows more? 4) check your internal moral compass.

6. What are the differences between informational social influence and normative social influence? What are social norms? Why are they followed so often?
    - normative social infl = need to be accepted.
    - social norms = rules a grp. has for acceptable behaviours, values, beliefs.
    - social norms are usu. followed to avoid ridicule, rejection.

7. Why were the findings of Asch's conformity study surprising? Were Asch's participants more likely conforming due to informational social influence or normative social influence? Explain.   - b/c task was obvious, unambiguous, people did not act rationally.
  - normative social infl. b/c. people knew were giving incorrect answers to avoid looking peculiar or odd. (public compliance).

8. According to Schachter's (1951) study, how do people deal with a nonconformist?

  - rejection, ostracize, assigned most boring, unimportant jobs.

9. What are historical examples of normative social influence? What do they tell us about the power and consequences of conforming due to social pressures?

  - raves; train "surfing" in Brazil; participating in beatings (eg. Reena Virk; (drugs)   (Can Airborne Regiment) ⟹ can be dangerous, deadly.

10. What does social impact theory attempt to explain? To what do the variables of strength, immediacy, and number of influence sources refer? What is the relationship between these variables and conformity?
  - that conforming to social infl. depends on the strength, immediacy, & numbers of a grp.
  - strength = importance of group, ie family, friends vs. strangers ⎫ - 3 more likely to conform
  - immediacy = how close in space & time a grp. is to you. ⎬ ⟹ however, less infl.
  - # = how many people in grp. ⎭ effect the larger the #

11. When will people conform due to normative social influence? What are the main ⟹ infl. by 3-4 conditions that increase this conformity?   vs. more.
  - as above, plus: when the group is unanimous, poss. personality & gender diffs, collectivist vs. independent cultural diffs.

12. What are cross-cultural differences in conformity? Has conformity increased or decreased since the 1950's?

  - similar today per Schachter's 1951 study. p. 281; similar examples today.

13. Do personality traits readily predict who will conform due to normative social influence? Why or why not?
  - conflicting evidence.

14. What is the magnitude of sex differences in influencibility? Under what conditions are women more likely to conform than men? Why?
  - small tendency for women to conform more than men, esp. in group-pressure
  - situations b/c gender roles dictate that men socialized to be individualists while women socialized to be cooperative.

15. What are two steps toward nonconformity? What are idiosyncrasy credits?

    - Find an ally or allies
    - act of conforming allows idiosyncrasy credits, to allow occasional deviant behaviour w/o retribution.

16. What are important conditions for the occurrence of minority influence? How do minorities tend to influence majorities? What is more likely a result of minority influence, public compliance or private acceptance?

    - consistency, others in minority must agree.
    - exert infl. thru informational social infl. ⇒ causing grp to examine issues carefully.

17. What is the relationship between the door-in-the-face technique and the reciprocity norm? - pressures us to reciprocate by moderating our position: from large refusal to smaller, reasonable response.

    - by receiving small "gift", must reciprocate.

18. Why is the foot-in-the-door technique effective?

    - effective b/c changes one's self-perception as a "giving" or "helpful" person.

19. What are the basic findings of the Milgram obedience study? What percentage of participants delivered the highest voltage of shock possible? Why was it difficult for participants in Milgram's studies to disobey authority? How do informational social influence and normative social influence help us understand Milgram's findings?

    - 65% complied & gave max. amt. of shock possible
    - b/c normative & informational social influence ⇒ pressure from authority figure; sit'n = unfamiliar & confusing, relied on "expert" for guidance.

20. What do variations of Milgram's study tell us about limits to obedience to authority?

    - obedience drops when others (allies) model disobedience & when "expert" not present.
    - w/no specific orders, almost no-one gives shocks.

PRACTICE QUIZ CHAPTER 8

Fill-in-the-Blank

1. A change in behaviour due to the real or imagined influence of other people is called

   _____.

2. An influence to conform to other people's behaviour because it defines an ambiguous situation for us and helps us choose appropriate courses of action is called

   _____.

3. Conforming to other people's behaviour out of a genuine belief that what they are doing or saying is right is called _____.

4.   Conforming to other people's behaviour publicly, without necessarily believing in what you are doing or saying is called _____.

5.   The rapid transmission of emotions or behaviour through a crowd is called _____.

6.   Implicit or explicit rules a group has for the acceptable behaviours, values, and beliefs of its members are called _____.

7.   An influence to conform to other people's behaviour in order to be liked or accepted by others is called _____.

8   A technique to induce compliance whereby people are presented with a large request and are expected to refuse it, and then presented with a smaller request is called the _____.

9.   A social norm which dictates that we should do something nice for someone who has done something nice for us is called the _____.

10.   A theory which states that conformity to social influence depends on the strength, immediacy, and number of others in the group is known as _____.

11.   The credits a person earns, over time, by conforming to group norms are called _____.

12.   The effect that a minority of group members has on the behaviour or beliefs of the majority is called _____.

13.   The compliance technique whereby people are first asked a small request and then are asked a larger one is called the _____.

Multiple Choice

14.   Why did individual estimates of a light's apparent motion converge when participants in Sherif's (1951) experiment called out their estimates in a group?
a)   Because participants used each other as a source of information.
b)   Because participants wanted to be liked by the others.
c)   Because participants badgered each other until everyone agreed.
d)   Because the mere presence of others had subtle effects on participants' visual processes.

15. Which of the following are recommended steps for resisting informational social influence?
    a)   Remember that resistance is possible and determine the sensibility of the available information.
    b)   Remember that unanimous majorities are rarely wrong and determine the strength of agreement within the majority.
    c)   Remember that people's opinions differ and search out advice from a similar individual.
    d)   Remember that you can't please everybody and that membership in some groups is more important than membership in others.

16. How was Asch's conformity study different from Sherif's?
    a)   Asch created an ambiguous situation while Sherif created an unambiguous one.
    b)   Asch created an unambiguous situation while Sherif created an ambiguous one.
    c)   The subjects in Asch's study were better problem-solvers than those in Sherif's study.
    d)   Accomplices in Asch's study imposed greater pressure on participants than did accomplices in Sherif's study.

17. When participants in Asch's (1956) study indicated which of three comparison lines matched a standard line by writing their responses on a piece of paper rather than by saying them out loud, conformity
    a)   increased somewhat.
    b)   remained the same.
    c)   dropped dramatically.
    d)   dropped slightly.

18. While stopped at a traffic light in a large city, a man appears from nowhere and, without asking, sprays your windshield with cleaner and wipes off the glass. The man realises that you are likely to tip him if you, like most people, obey the ____ norm.
    a)   generosity
    b)   morality
    c)   obedience
    d)   reciprocity

19. According to Latane's (1981) social impact theory, the amount of influence that people whose opinions differ from your own will exert will be greatest if they are in a group that is
    a)   comprised of 3 people.
    b)   important.
    c)   unanimous.
    d)   b and c

20. Replications of Asch's (1956) conformity research across many cultures and different time periods indicate that amounts of conformity
    a)   are constant culture to culture and over time in a given culture.
    b)   vary from culture to culture but are constant over time in a given culture.
    c)   vary from culture to culture and over time in a given culture.
    d)   are constant culture to culture but vary over time in a given culture.

21. Which of the following most accurately summarises research on individual differences in conformity?
    a)   an individual's personality traits predict conformity over a wide range of situations but gender is a poor predictor of conformity.
    b)   personality traits and gender may account for small differences in conformity but the relationship between these and conformity is not clear-cut.
    c)   women conform to a much greater extent than do men but personality traits that reliably predict conformity have not been found.
    d)   both personality traits and gender predict conformity over a wide range of situations.

22. The first step in resisting normative social influence is to
    a)   ignore the source of influence.
    b)   take action to avoid being influenced.
    c)   find an ally to assist in resisting influence.
    d)   become aware of the norms guiding behaviour.

23. In Milgram's obedience studies participants played the role of "teacher" in what they believed was an experiment on the effects of punishment on learning. Throughout the experiment they feared they might kill a "learner" with increasingly higher electrical shocks. Mild prods by an authority to "please continue" were nonetheless enough to get ___% of Milgram's participants to obey completely.
    a)   1.0
    b)   12.5
    c)   36.0
    d)   62.5

24. Which of the following forms of social influence induced the participants in Milgram's obedience studies to administer the maximum level of shock possible to a helpless learner?
    a)   normative social influence
    b)   informational social influence
    c)   both normative and informational social influence
    d)   neither normative nor informational social influence

25. Conformity is
    a)   the spread of emotions and behaviours throughout a large group.
    b)   the occurrence of similar physical symptoms in a group of people with no known physical cause.
    c)   a rule for acceptable social behaviour.
    d)   a change in behaviour due to the real or imagined influence of other people.

26. Whereas normative social influence leads to _____, informational social influence produces _____.
   a) private acceptance; public compliance
   b) public compliance; private acceptance
   c) conformity; minority influence
   d) minority influence; conformity

27. Asch (1956) presented participants with three comparison lines and a standard line that clearly matched one of the comparison lines. When participants were asked to publicly identify the matching line they went along with a rigged majority and made incorrect judgements
   a) almost every time.
   b) about half of the time.
   c) about a third of the time.
   d) almost never.

28. Bibb Latane's social impact (1981) theory describes
   a) characteristics that make a source influential.
   b) the type of people who are most likely to conform.
   c) when conformity is foolish and when it is wise.
   d) cognitive processes involved in "mindless" conformity.

29. Personality traits have been found to be poor predictors of conformity because
   a) the social situation is often as important in understanding how someone will behave as is his or her personality.
   b) personality traits that might influence conformity have not been identified.
   c) gender is often as important in understanding how someone will behave as is his or her personality.
   d) all of the above

30. Alice Eagly (1987) believes that women may exhibit more conforming behaviour than men only when an audience is present because
   a) women are less confident of themselves in front of an audience than men.
   b) women are more easily influenced than men.
   c) women are less socially adept than men.
   d) gender roles dictate that men should be individualists while women should be cooperative.

31. The reciprocity norm has been linked with which of the following compliance techniques?
   a) the foot-in-the-face technique
   b) the door-in-the-face technique
   c) the foot-in-the-door technique
   d) minority influence technique

32.   Why did obedience by participants in Milgram's studies drop drastically when two accomplices, acting as fellow teachers, refused to obey the experimenter?
        a)   Because the participant could not continue without the help of the accomplice teachers.
        b)   Because similar peers exert more normative social influence than do dissimilar authority figures.
        c)   Because the accomplices served as allies which enabled participants to resist normative social influence.
        d)   Because the two accomplices outnumbered the experimenter and formed an influential majority.

Short Essay

33.   Give three reasons why participants obeyed the experimenter in Milgram's studies.

34.   Make two columns with the headings "informational social influence" and "normative social influence". List the following names and terms under the appropriate heading: Asch, Schachter, Milgram, Sherif, minority influence, "mindless" conformity, contagion.

35.   Compare and contrast normative and informational social influence. Why are they called "social" influence? What motives underlie each type of influence and what effects does each type have on our behaviour?

36.   Why is Asch's conformity study "one of the most dramatic illustrations of blindly going along with the group, even when the individual realises that by doing so he turns his back on reality and truth"? (Moscovici, 1985, p. 349)

37.   Describe Bibb Latane's (1981) Social Impact Theory. What are the sources of social impact and what characteristics of these sources determine the amount of impact a group will have?

CHAPTER 9

Group Processes: Influence in Social Groups

CHAPTER OVERVIEW

Chapter 9 considers how groups influence the behaviours of their members. Groups exist in a wide variety of forms. Groups are defined in the first section of this chapter. Social facilitation, social loafing, and deindividuation are then considered. Social loafing and social facilitation are closely related. Arousal due to the presence of others can facilitate or hinder our performance. The complexity of the task also must be considered. This section outlines these corresponding conditions. Deindividuation helps explain the behaviour of people in large groups when they feel anonymous and unaccountable for their actions.

The next section discusses research on group decision-making. Process loss and group polarization are reviewed. Leadership theories are also addressed in this section. Two theories concerned with leadership effectiveness are examined. The last section of this chapter focuses on conflict and cooperation. The phenomenon of social dilemmas is explored. Conditions that foster trust and cooperation are discussed.

CHAPTER OUTLINE

Definitions: What Is a Group?

>   Why Do People Join Groups?

>   The Composition of Groups

How Groups Influence the Behaviour of Individuals

>   Social Facilitation: When the Presence of Others Energizes Us

>   Social Loafing: When the Presence of Others Relaxes Us

>   Deindividuation: Getting Lost in the Crowd

Group Decisions: Are Two (or More) Heads Better than One?

>   Process Loss: When Group Interactions Inhibit Good Problem Solving

>   Group Polarization: Going to Extremes

>   Leadership in Groups

Conflict and Cooperation

>   Social Dilemmas

>   Using Threats to Resolve Conflict

>   Negotiation and Bargaining

LEARNING OBJECTIVES

After reading Chapter 9, you should be able to do the following:

1. Provide a definition of groups and discuss why people join groups. Distinguish social roles, social norms and gender roles. Discuss the composition of groups and define group cohesiveness. (pp. 305-310)

2. Define social facilitation. Explain why the presence of others causes arousal. Discuss the effects of social facilitation on the performance of simple and complex tasks. (pp. 310-315)

3. Describe social loafing and discuss why it occurs. Identify how the setting in which social loafing occurs is different from the setting in which social facilitation occurs. Identify gender and cultural differences that increase and decrease social loafing. (pp. 315-317)

4. Define deindividuation and describe the effects of deindividuation on behaviour. Identify conditions that increase deindividuation. (pp. 317-320)

5. Identify sources of process loss in groups. Describe how group members handle unique information during discussion. Identify how groups could improve the sharing of information. (pp. 320-323)

6. Identify the antecedents, symptoms, and consequences of groupthink. Discuss historical examples of groupthink. Identify measures that can be taken to avoid groupthink. (pp. 323-325)

7. Describe the effects of group discussion on attitudes that are initially risky or initially cautious. Describe the persuasive arguments and social comparison explanations for group polarization. (pp. 325-327)

8. Describe the relationship between the great person theory and great leadership. Identify the personality traits and variables that are related to leadership. Contrast the great person theory with the contingency theory of leadership. Identify the different types of leaders according to the contingency theory. Discuss the relationship between gender and leadership. (pp. 327-332)

9. Describe the type of conflict known as a social dilemma. Describe the prisoner's dilemma. Identify the tit-for-tat strategy and describe why it is effective. (pp. 332-335)

10. Describe the consequences of using threats to address conflict. Describe conditions when communication facilitates cooperation. (pp. 335-338)

11. Identify effective negotiation strategies. Describe an integrative solution. Identify obstacles to finding integrative solutions. (pp. 338-340)

KEY TERMS

STUDY QUESTIONS

1. Define roles and the function of roles in social groups.
    - shared expectations in a grp. about how particular people are supposed to behave
    - helpful b/c people know what to expect from ea. other.
        ⟹ people will tend to be satisfied & perform well.

2.   What are the conditions that facilitate social facilitation effects? What role does task difficulty play in social facilitation effects? How and why does arousal interact with task difficulty when people are performing a task in the presence of others?

     1) presence of others increases physiological arousal (energizes us).
     2) w/ arousal, easier to do simple tasks (dominant responses) rather than new or complex tasks.
     2) when individual performance can be evaluated.
   B/C ⟹ 1) presence of others makes us alert; 2) "evaluation apprehension"; 3) distraction by others

3.   What are the conditions that facilitate social loafing effects? What are effective ways to reduce social loafing?

     1) presence of others
     2) performance cannot be evaluated. } ⟹ do worse on simple tasks, better on complex tasks.

     — use of computers for anonymous interaction, but w/ safeguards.

4.   What implications do social facilitation and social loafing have for organising groups in work situations?

     — for simple tasks, evaluation apprehension shud improve performance.
     — for complex tasks, lowered evaluation apprehension by placing inds in grps where indiv perf. can not be observed will improve perf.

5.   What is deindividuation? What behaviours does it help to explain? Why does deindividuation happen?

     — loosening of normal constraints on behaviour in a grp situation, which leads to an increase in impulsive & deviant acts.
     — greater aggression, violence
     — presence of others decreases accountability; lowers self-awareness (ignore moral stds.)

6.   Why do people join groups? What are the benefits of social group membership? What are group roles and what functions do they serve? What are possible costs to social roles?

     — help us define who we are, identity; motivates us to become involved in social change; innate → food, children, mating.
     — can "lose" identity/personality if take on role too much; acting inconsistent w/ established roles can lead to ostracization & rejection.

7.   What is the great person theory and what does it attempt to predict and explain?

     — key personality traits make a person a good leader, regardless of the situation.
     — shud be able to isolate traits to predict a good leader, eg. charisma, intelligence, courage etc.,

8.   According to the contingency theory of leadership, what are two types of leaders? Under what conditions is each type of leader most effective?

     — relationship-oriented: concerned w/ feelings of/ships b/n workers ⟹ best when situational control= moderate
     — task-oriented: concerned w/ getting job done ⟹ best when situational control is high or low

9.   What do research findings tell us about gender differences in leadership effectiveness?

     — women lead more democratically, better interpersonal skills, but can be assertive when necessary
       ⟹ altho this is viewed negatively by others, particularly males

10. What is process loss in groups? How does it occur?

- any aspect of grp. interaction that inhibits good problem solving.
- by not trying to find most competent member; narrative conformity pressure on most competent member; comm. probs; failing to discuss info that other members do not know.

11. What is groupthink? What are its symptoms? How can it be avoided?

- thinking that maintains grp. cohesiveness & solidarity over considering the facts in a realistic manner.
- occurs when grp = highly cohesive, isolated from contrary opinions, views of leader known; high stress; poor decision-making strategies. Symptoms = illusion of invulnerability; belief in moral correctness of grp; stereotyped views

12. What is group polarization? How does it happen?

of outgrp; self-censorship; pressure on others to conform; illusion unanimity; mindguards;
- tendency for grps to make decisions that are more extreme than initial inclinations of ind. grp. members.
⇒ leadershud remain impartial, invite outside opinions, create subgroups; secret ballots.
1) persuasive argument interpretation - consider other views.
2) social comparison interpretation - take pos. sim. to others value.

13. What is a social dilemma? What is the tit-for-tat strategy? When is it best to use this strategy in the prisoner's dilemma game?

- conflict in which beneficial action for an individual may have overall harmful effects to others.
- encouraging cooperation by 1st acting cooperatively, & then responding in kind to opponent.
- best to encourage cooperation & trust.

14. Are threats an effective means to reduce conflict? Explain. When can communication alleviate conflict?

- NO - when threatened by force, opponents will retaliate ⇒ produces stalemates.
- comm. can alleviate if instructed to be fair, & imagine self in others shoes.

15. What strategies do people use when they negotiate? Which strategies are most successful for reducing conflict? What is an integrative solution and what are barriers to these solutions?

- talking, bargaining, making counteroffers until both parties agree.
- find solutions favourable to both parties.
⇒ make trade-offs according to diff. interests - concede on issues unimportant to you but not to the other party; however, diff. to discover opponents true interests, altho. believe shud be obvious.

PRACTICE QUIZ CHAPTER 9

Fill-in-the-Blank

1. Arousal which results from other people's physical and evaluative presence and which enhances performance on simple tasks but impairs performance on complex tasks is called _____.

2. Relaxation and the reduction of individual effort which results when the performance of group members cannot be evaluated is called _____.

3. The loosening of normal constraints on behaviour, leading to an increase in impulsive and deviant acts, is called _____.

4. Any aspect of group interaction that inhibits good problem solving is known as _____.

5. A kind of thinking in which maintaining group cohesiveness and solidarity is more important than considering the facts in a realistic manner is called _____.

6. The tendency for groups to make decisions that are more extreme than the initial inclinations of its members is called _____.

7. The theory that leadership effectiveness depends on how task-oriented or relationship-oriented the leader is and on how much control over the group the leader has is called the _____ theory of leadership.

8. A leader who is concerned mostly with how well workers are getting along is a _____ leader.

9. The theory that certain personality traits make a person an effective leader is called the _____ theory.

10. A means of encouraging cooperation by acting cooperatively at first , and then by matching the (cooperative or competitive) responses of one's opponent on subsequent trials, is called the _____ strategy.

11. A form of communication between opposing sides in a conflict, in which offers and counteroffers are made and a solution occurs only when it is agreed on by both parties, is called _____.

12. A solution to a conflict that finds outcomes favourable to both parties is called a(n) _____.

13. _____ is the combined memory of two people.

14. A conflict in which the best action for one person if chosen by everyone will harm everyone is called a _____.

Multiple Choice

15. If you are asked to perform in the presence of others, you are likely to feel aroused as a result of
    a) anticipatory arousal.
    b) increased interpersonal conflict.
    c) increased alertness and evaluation apprehension.
    d) disinhibition.

16. Compared to individuals, members of social loafing groups perform ____ on simple tasks and ____ on complex tasks.
    a) better; worse
    b) worse; better
    c) worse; worse
    d) better; better

17. To maximise the performance of seasoned workers performing familiar tasks at your production plant, you should create groups that foster _____.
   a) social loafing
   b) social facilitation
   c) deindividuation
   d) conflict

18. Groups that strengthen the initial inclinations of their members, pushing their members' decisions to the extreme, exhibit _____.
   a) the risky shift
   b) social facilitation
   c) process loss
   d) group polarization

19. Integrative solutions to conflicts are most likely to be reached if
   a) opponents find out which issues being negotiated are most important to each party.
   b) opponents compromise on all issues being negotiated.
   c) negotiations are arbitrated by a neutral third party.
   d) communication between opponents is limited to a structured exchange of ideas.

20. Zajonc et al. (1969) observed that cockroaches took longer to reach a dark box at the end of a maze when other cockroaches were present if
   a) the maze was a simple one.
   b) the maze was a complex one.
   c) the other cockroaches first modelled the escape behaviour.
   d) the other cockroaches served as a source of evaluation.

21. In order to know whether the presence of others will improve a group member's performance or hinder it, you need to know
   a) whether the individual can be evaluated and whether the task is simple or complex.
   b) whether group members interact and whether the goals of group members conflict.
   c) whether the members of the group are disposed to be lazy and whether the group will be tightly organised.
   d) how much communication among members is possible and how well members of the group get along.

22. A social dilemma is a situation which may result in a conflict because
   a) people work harder in groups than they do when working alone.
   b) individuals may seek to maximise personal gain at the expense of others.
   c) process loss results when individuals are in a social situation
   d) individuals make better decisions than groups do

23. European soccer fans attacking each other and hysterical fans at rock concerts trampling one another to death demonstrate the horrendous consequences of ____.
    a)   social facilitation
    b)   group polarization
    c)   deindividuation
    d)   interpersonal conflict

24. Which of the following proposes that leadership effectiveness can be predicted by traits that people may or may not possess?
    a)   the contingency theory of leadership
    b)   the integrative theory of leadership
    c)   the great person theory of leadership
    d)   the process theory of leadership

25. In which situations are task-oriented leaders more effective than relationship-oriented leaders?
    a)   when situational control is moderate
    b)   when workers get along fairly well
    c)   when the task is somewhat structured
    d)   when situational control is high

26. According to persuasive arguments interpretation, group polarization results because
    a)   individuals bring to the group strong and novel arguments supporting their initial inclinations.
    b)   group discussion reveals the position that the group values and individuals adopt this position in order to be liked.
    c)   individuals recognise that western culture values risk over caution.
    d)   groups actively censor opinions that deviate from those valued by our culture.

27. Initially choosing a cooperative response, and then matching your opponent's response on subsequent trials is an effective strategy in mixed-motive games called ____.
    a)   dog-eat-dog
    b)   acquiescence
    c)   integrative solutions
    d)   tit-for-tat

28. A crowd committing terrible crimes than few individuals would do on their own can best be explained through the process of
    a)   groupthink
    b)   deindividuation
    c)   social loafing
    d)   social facilitation

29. During group discussion, group members tend to focus on the information that
    a)   all group members share
    b)   is held by a few members
    c)   is irrelevant to the task at hand
    d)   cannot be known before the decision is made

30.   Deutsch and Krauss (1960) found that when participants in the trucking game had the opportunity to communicate with each other but were not required to do so,
a)   performance improved substantially
b)   few participants communicated
c)   communication was irrelevant to the task at hand
d)   trust between participants increased

Short Essay

31.   What is group polarization? Discuss the role of cognitive and motivational factors in producing group polarization.

32.   Riots and other instances of unruly mob behaviour are the result of what group process? What characteristics of the group and situation combine to produce such negative behaviours?

33.   Describe several causes, symptoms, and consequences of groupthink.

34.   What is negotiation? Describe effective negotiation strategies. What strategies are likely to be helpful when negotiations break down?

CHAPTER 10

Interpersonal Attraction: From First Impressions to Close Relationships

CHAPTER OVERVIEW

Chapter 10 examines the causes of liking and loving that have been studied. The factors which contribute to liking are revealed in the first section of this chapter. We like people who are familiar to us, physically attractive, similar to us, and who like us.

The next section of the chapter tackles the complexities of defining love. Two theories have conceptualized love by defining its types. A common distinction is made between passionate love and companionate love. A third conception of love states that people are guided in close relationships by their love styles. Six love styles are identified. Cultural differences in beliefs about what is important in a marriage partner are also addressed.

The causes of love are examined next. Evolutionary theory offers explanations of topics such as gender differences in mate selection. Research on attachment styles has shown to be useful in understanding the dynamics of close relationships. Social exchange theories predict relationships will develop when there is the possibility of a mutually beneficial exchange.

Next, factors that predict whether relationships will be maintained are discussed. Social exchange theory is again examined in addition to the role of adversity and positive illusions in relationship maintenance. Sadly, many relationships are not happy and do not last. Strategies people use in response to relationship problems and the consequences of role in the dissolution process are examined.

CHAPTER OUTLINE

Major Antecedents of Attraction

      The Person Next Door: The Propinquity Effect

      Similarity

      Reciprocal Liking

      The Effects of Physical Attractiveness on Liking

Forming Close Relationships: Defining Love

      What is Love?

      Gender and Love

      Culture and Love

LEARNING OBJECTIVES

After reading Chapter 10, you should be able to do the following:

1. Describe the role of propinquity in attraction. Distinguish between physical and functional distance. Explain how the propinquity effect works. (pp. 347-350)

2. Discuss the importance of similarity in attraction. Identify why we like people whose characteristics and beliefs are similar to our own. (pp. 350-351)

3. Discuss the importance of reciprocal liking in attraction. Discuss the role of self-esteem in reciprocal liking. (p. 351)

4. Discuss the consequences of physical attractiveness for liking strangers and for maintaining relationships. Identify the facial features associated with high attractiveness in females and in males. (pp. 352-355)

5. Discuss how perceptions of attractiveness is similar across cultures. Describe the "what is beautiful is good" stereotype and explain how this stereotype might produce a self-fulfilling prophecy. Discuss support for the notion that "beauty is in the eye of the beholder." (pp. 355-359)

6. Distinguish between passionate and companionate types of love proposed by Hatfield. Identify the combinations of intimacy, passion, and commitment that produce the various types of love outlined in Sternberg's triangular theory of love. (pp. 359-362)

7. Define the six styles of love according to Hendrick and Hendrick. Differentiate social psychologists' and ordinary people's definitions of love. (pp. 362-364)

8. Discuss gender and cultural differences in how people label the experiences of romantic love and in how they make decisions to marry. Identify cultural differences in love styles. (pp. 364-367)

9. Describe evolutionary biology's explanation of the experience of romantic love. (pp. 367-368)

10. Identify the key assumption of attachment theory and distinguish between the three attachment styles. Discuss support for attachment theory in intimate relationships. (pp. 368-372)

11. Describe social exchange theory. Identify the basic concepts of social exchange theory. Distinguish between comparison level and comparison level for alternatives. (pp. 372-373)

12. Describe equity theory and indicate how partners in a relationship respond when they are over- or underbenefited in an inequitable relationship. Identify how equity theory differs from social exchange theory. (pp. 373-374)

13. Discuss support for social exchange theory in long-term intimate relationships. Describe the relationship between social exchange theory and Rusbult's investment model. Identify what things we need to know in order to predict whether people will stay in an intimate relationship. (pp. 374-376)

14. Describe how partners' concerns with equity differ depending on whether the partners are involved in an exchange or in a communal relationship. (pp. 376-377)

15. Discuss the role of adversity in maintaining relationships. What role doe positive illusions play in relationship maintenance? (pp. 378-381)

16. Discuss research findings in the area of relationship ending. (pp. 381-383)

KEY TERMS

propinquity effect (p. 347)

mere exposure effect (p. 348)

similarity (p. 350)

complementarity (p. 350)

reciprocal liking (p. 351)

companionate love (p. 360)

passionate love (p. 360)

triangular theory of love (p. 361)

love styles (p. 362)

evolutionary approach (p. 367)

attachment styles (p. 369)

secure attachment style (p. 369)

avoidant attachment style (p. 369)

anxious/ambivalent attachment style (p. 369)

fearful avoidant style (p. 370)

dismissive avoidant style (p. 370)

social exchange theory (p. 372)

reward/cost ratio (p. 373)

comparison level (p. 373)

comparison level for alternatives (p. 373)

equity theory (p. 373)

investment model (p. 375)

exchange relationships (p. 376)

communal relationships (p. 376)

commitment calibration hypothesis (p. 378)

positive illusions (p. 380)

STUDY QUESTIONS

1. What is the relationship between propinquity and attraction? What is the mere exposure effect?
   - the more we see & interact w/ people, the more likely they will be our friends.
   - work b/c of familiarity or the "mere-exposure" effect: the more exposure we have to a stimulus, the more apt we are to like it. (same for the converse → dislike).

2. Why is similarity such an important factor in attraction?
   - attraction to people who are like us (demographically, attitudes, values etc, activity preferences) b/c believe those similar will like us (→ more inclined to initiate r'ship), will validate our characteristics & beliefs, will feel more understood, & the desire for enjoyable interactions (à la the "rewards-of-interaction" explanation).

3. Why is reciprocal liking important in attraction?
   - liking someone who likes us in return = prime determinant of interpersonal attraction.
   - can make up for absence of similarity
   - can come about b/c of self-fulfilling prophecy (but only if you like yourself in the first place → neg. self-concepts = skeptical).

4. What are the effects of physical attractiveness on liking? What are facial features associated with high attractiveness in females and in males? What are cross-cultural findings on the perceptions of physical attractiveness?
   - overriding determinant on liking → altho don't like to admit it; best predictor of desirability.
   - greater emph. on looks for men.
   - facial features = small noses, big eyes, high cheekbones, shapely lips, clear skin, (slim bodies) (athletic)
     - females = high eyebrows, big smile, small chin, narrow cheeks
     - males = large chin, big smile. } cultural similarity (agreement) for attractive faces ⇒ arithmetic means.

5. What stereotypes are associated with physical attractiveness? What role does the self-fulfilling prophecy play in the perpetuation of these assumptions? What are cross-cultural findings regarding the "what is beautiful is good" stereotype?
   - "what is beautiful is good" stereotype = physical attractiveness is highly correlated w/ desirable traits.
   - for older men, " = younger, for women. ⇒ usu. social competence.
   - attractive people, from a young age receive more social attn which helps develop good social skills → leads to interpersonal/occupational success.
   - cross-culturally = similar stereotype; however, also value integrity: concern for others' traits vs. independence, self reliance traits of indi. culture.

6. How does the social exchange theory explain how people feel about their relationships? What are comparisons that people make according to this theory?
   - how one feels about r'ships depends on one's perceptions of the rewards & costs of the r'ship, the kind of r'ship one thinks deserves, & their chances of having a better r'ship w/ another. ⇒ reward, cost, outcome, comparison level, comparison level for alternatives.
   - comparison level = expectations re: the level of rewards & costs they deserve in r'ships - (history)
   - " " for alternatives = expectations re: level of rewards & costs wd receive in another r'ship. high = more likely to leave current r'ship, low = likely to stay in costly r'ship

7. What accounts for happy relationships according to equity theory?
   - r'ships in which rewards & costs that one experiences & the contributions one makes are roughly equal to the rewards, costs, & contributions of the other person. = most happy & stable.

8. What are differences between companionate love and passionate love?
   - companionate love = feelings of intimacy & affection we feel about some we care deeply for (eg. family, friends; but also sexual r'ships (w/o passion).
   - passionate love = intense longing & physiological arousal we feel for another - when reciprocated = fulfillment & ecstasy; when not, sadness & despair. (characterized by obsessive thots, heightened arousal when near the person).

comparionate love.

Intimacy

Romantic / *cons.* *Compationate*

Passionate *Commitment*

Fatuous

9. **What are the three basic ingredients of love according to the triangular theory of love? What are the types of love formed by varying degrees of these ingredients?**

all = consummate love.

{ - intimacy, passion, commitment   Intimacy & commitment

romantic love   Fatuous love   Compationate love

10. **How do the six styles of love differ from each other? What roles do gender and culture play in the endorsement of the different love styles?**
    1) Eros = passionate, physical   5) Mania = emotional, roller coaster: obsess: elation/despair
    2) Ludus = playful game, not serious 6) Agape = selfless, giving, altruistic.
    3) Storge = slow-growing, evolving from f'ship ⇒ men more romantic; women more practical
    4) Pragma = realistic, commonsensical ⇒ asian (collectivist) = more storgic.

11. **How does culture influence both the definition of love and the behaviours that correspond with it?**
    - collectivist cultures value compationate love more, takes into acct. wishes of family & friends, arranged marriages.
    - individualist cultures value passionate love, personal experience, ignores others -

12. **What does the social exchange theory help explain in the area of long-term relationships?**
    - will be happy in r'ship as long as rewards outweigh costs. Reward/cost ratios must exceed our comparison level. Also, if we don't have attractive alternatives available.

    - However, need to consider

13. **What are the postulates of the investment model? What is the definition of investments according to this model?**
    - commit to r'ship depends on satisfaction w/r'ship in terms of rewards, costs, & comparison level; comparison level for alternatives; & how much invested in r'ship wld be lost by leaving it.   (tangibles)   (intangibles)
    - investments = financial resources/possessions; emotional welfare of kids, time & energy spent on r'ship

14. **How do exchange relationships differ from communal relationships?**
    - exchange = r'ships governed by need for equity ⇒ comparable ratio of rewards & cost (tit-for-tat strategy ⇒ casual r'ships).
    - communal = r'ships where primary concern is being responsive to others' needs ⇒ desire to help others regardless of repayment, relaxed re: equity, believe will balance over time.

15. **What are the major tenets of evolutionary theory as it relates to love? What are other explanations for gender differences in mate selection?**   (eg. parenting close friends, family romantic partners
    - biological reproductive success depends on 2 diff. behaviour patterns: men attracted to appearance, women attracted to resources to maximize reproductive success.
    - men conditioned to value physical attractiveness & youth ⇒ media; w/economic power, women seek same qualities (conscious).

16. **How do attachment styles develop and how do they manifest themselves in later relationships? What do people with each style report about their relationships?**
    - attachment styles develop based on our experiences as infants w/ our primary caregiver.
    ⇒ secure = caregivers responsive & positive to needs, not worried re: abandoned, feel worthy & loved ⇒ easily close to others, trusting, satisfying r'ships.
    ⇒ avoidant = aloof, distant caregivers, rebuff attempts for intimacy ⇒ uncomfortable becoming close to others, distrusting, less satisfying r'ships -
    ⇒ anxious/ambivalent = inconsistent or overbearing in affection caregivers ⇒ fear partners do not desire to be close/intimate w/ them, obsessive & unsatisfying r'ships.

17. What are four basic endings to romantic relationships according to people's accounts of their breakups?

   - withdrawal/avoidance (passive); positive tone; manipulative strategies (3rd party); open confrontation.

18. What is perhaps the most important predictor of psychological and physical effects of relationship dissolution? What is the best way to end a relationship? What determines whether people will remain friends after their relationship ends?

   - breaker vs. breakee max distressed.   => confrontation for romantic r'ships.
   - mutual = mutually distressing.

PRACTICE QUIZ CHAPTER 10

Fill-in-the-Blank

1. The finding that the more we see and interact with people, the more likely they are to become our friends is called the _____.

2. The finding that the more exposure we have to a stimulus, the more apt we are to like it is called _____.

3. The basic ideas people have about love that influence their behaviour are called _____.

4. How people feel about a relationship depends on their perceptions of the rewards and costs of the relationship, the kind of relationship they deserve, and their chances for having a better relationship with someone else. This is the rationale of _____ theory.

5. People's expectations about the level of rewards and punishments they are likely to receive in a particular relationship comprise their _____.

6. People's expectations about the level of rewards and punishments they would receive in an alternative relationship comprise their

   _____.

7. People are happiest with relationships in which the rewards, costs, and contributions of one person in a relationship roughly equal the rewards, costs, and contributions of the other person in the relationship. This is the rationale of _____ theory.

8. The feelings of intimacy and affection we feel toward someone that are not accompanied by passion or physiological arousal are called _____.

9. The feelings of intense longing for another person accompanied by physiological arousal are called _____.

10. The theory that states different kinds of love consist of varying degrees intimacy, passion, and commitment is called the _____.

11. People's commitment to a relationship depends on their satisfaction with the relationship, their comparison level for alternatives, and their level of investment in the relationship. This is the rationale of the _____.

12. Relationships governed by the need for equity are called _____ relationships.

13. Relationships in which people's primary concern is being responsive to the other person's needs are called _____ relationships.

14. The expectations people develop about relationships with others, based on the relationship they had with their primary caregiver when they were infants, characterise their _____.

15. An attachment style characterised by trust, a lack of concern with being abandoned, and the view that one is worthy and well liked is called a(n) _____ attachment style.

16. An attachment style characterised by a suppression of attachment needs and by difficulty developing intimate relationships is known as a(n) _____ attachment style.

17. An attachment style characterised by a concern that others will not reciprocate one's desire for intimacy, resulting in higher-than-average levels of anxiety is called a (n) _____ attachment style.

18. According to the _____ hypothesis, adversity can strengthen a relationship only if commitment and adversity are equal.

Multiple Choice

19. When you were eight years old, chances are you were best friends with someone who lived on your block. Social psychologists would attribute this to
    a)   the effects of attitude similarity.
    b)   your uniquely similar interests.
    c)   matched levels of physical attractiveness.
    d)   the propinquity effect.

20. In their study of "blind dates," Elaine Hatfield and her colleagues (1966) found that an individual's desire to date his or her partner again was best predicted by the partner's
    a)   physical attractiveness.
    b)   dominance and sensitivity.
    c)   complementary personality traits.
    d)   intelligence.

21. Research has found all of the following facial features to be considered physically attractive EXCEPT
    a) large eyes.
    b) wide cheeks
    c) big smile
    d) small nose

22. Social exchange theory maintains that people are happiest with relationships when
    a) the perceived rewards of the relationship are equal to the perceived costs of the relationship.
    b) the rewards and costs a person experiences are roughly equal to the rewards and costs of the other person in a relationship.
    c) the actual rewards and costs of the relationship exceed the expected rewards and costs.
    d) the perceived rewards of the relationship outweigh the perceived costs of the relationship.

23. When the rewards and costs a person experiences and the contributions he/she makes to the relationship are roughly equal to the rewards, costs, and contributions of the other person, the relationship is _____.
    a) equitable
    b) communal
    c) intimate
    d) passionate

24. In Sternberg's triangular theory of love, consummate love is characterised by
    a) high levels of passion and low levels of commitment and intimacy.
    b) high levels of passion, commitment, and intimacy.
    c) high levels of commitment and passion and low levels of intimacy.
    d) high levels of passion and intimacy and low levels of commitment.

25. People are likely to remain committed to an intimate relationship even if they are dissatisfied with it and even if alternative relationships look promising if
    a) they suffer from low self-esteem.
    b) they have a high comparison level.
    c) they have benefited from the relationship in the past.
    d) they have invested heavily in the relationship.

26. In a happy communal relationship, partners believe that equity
    a) is of no importance.
    b) should exist at any given time.
    c) will be maintained in the long run.
    d) requires close monitoring at all times.

27. The ludic love style is characterised by
    a) intense longing for one's partner
    b) beliefs that love requires a long-term commitment
    c) beliefs that love is a game to be played
    d) beliefs that love develops from friendship

28. The desire to be validated and the conclusions we draw about people's characters based on their attitudes leads us to prefer people whose attitudes
   a) complement our own.
   b) are similar to our own.
   c) are generally positive.
   d) are well informed.

29. The comparison level for alternatives is based on
   a) perceptions of the level of rewards and punishments received from your primary caregiver during infancy.
   b) perceptions of the level of rewards and punishments others are receiving in their present relationships.
   c) expectations about the level of rewards and punishments others would receive if they were sharing a relationship with your partner.
   d) expectations about the level of rewards and punishments you would receive if you were in a different relationship.

30. A tit-for-tat equity norm governs _____ relationships.
   a) exchange
   b) communal
   c) familial
   d) romantic

31. Attachment styles are the expectations people develop about
   a) the level of rewards and punishments they are likely to receive in a particular relationship.
   b) the level of rewards and punishments they would receive in an alternative relationship.
   c) the kinds of actions by their partners that constitute a threat to their self-worth and produce feelings of jealousy.
   d) relationships with others based on the relationship they had with their primary caregiver when they were infants.

32. An individual who has an anxious/ambivalent attachment style
   a) finds it difficult to trust others and to develop close intimate relationships.
   b) is able to develop a mature, lasting relationship.
   c) wants to become very close to his/her partner but worries that his/her affections will not be returned.
   d) is not interested in developing a close relationship.

33. An approach which states that men are attracted by women's appearance and that women are attracted by men's resources is the:
   a) communal exchange theory
   b) investment model
   c) propinquity effect
   d) evolutionary approach to love

34. Which of the following is a style of love according to Hendrick and Hendrick?
    a)   mania
    b)   ludus
    c)   Eros
    d)   all of the above

35. An individual asked to picture a loved one for whom one has a secure relationship will be more attracted to a stranger who displays
    a)   a secure attachment style
    b)   an insecure attachment style
    c)   an avoidant attachment style
    d)   resistance to change

36. According to the commitment calibration hypothesis, efforts to preserve or maintain a relationship will occur only if the level of adversity in the relationship is
    a)   less than the level of commitment
    b)   equal to the level of commitment
    c)   greater than the level of commitment
    d)   unrelated to the level of commitment

Short Essay

37. What factors have been demonstrated to increase interpersonal attraction among casual acquaintances?

38. Identify facial features associated with attractiveness in men and in women. Describe the assumptions we make about attractive people and a consequence of making such assumptions.

39. Describe the key assumption of attachment theory. Describe the formation of each of the attachment styles in infancy and the consequences of each of these for adult relationships.

40. Define the six styles of love and gender and cultural differences in the endorsement of each style.

41. Compare and contrast social exchange theory with equity theory.

CHAPTER 11

Prosocial Behaviour: Why Do People Help?

CHAPTER OVERVIEW

In the first section of this chapter, you'll discover the three different motives that have been proposed to explain prosocial behaviour. The theory of evolutionary psychology, social exchange theory, and the empathy-altruism hypothesis each help us to understand why people help others. However, one of the difficulties of this research area is the complexity of distinguishing between behaviours motivated by self-interest and those that are truly altruistic.

The next section identifies the effects of individual differences such as personality, gender, culture, and mood on how likely people are to help in a variety of circumstances. Research topics on the altruistic personality, gender and cultural differences in the propensity to help in certain situations, and the conducive effects of both positive and negative moods on helping are examined. Situational determinants such as urban overload, the number of bystanders, and characteristics of the relationship, are discussed next. Latane and Darley's bystander intervention decision tree helps explain the several causes of the bystander effect. In the final section, strategies for increasing prosocial behaviour are developed from lessons learned throughout this chapter.

CHAPTER OUTLINE

Basic Motives Underlying Prosocial Behaviour

  Evolutionary Psychology: Instincts and Genes

  Social Exchange: The Costs and Rewards of Helping

  Empathy and Altruism: The Pure Motive for Helping

Personal Determinants of Prosocial Behaviour: Why Do Some People Help More than

Others?

  Individual Differences: The Altruistic Personality

  The Effects of Mood on Prosocial Behaviour

  Gender Differences in Prosocial Behaviour

  Cultural Differences in Prosocial Behaviour

Situational Determinants of Prosocial Behaviour: When Will People Help?

  Environment: Rural Versus Urban

Bystander Intervention: The Latane and Darley Model

The Nature of the Relationship: Communal Versus Exchange Relationships

How Can Helping Be Increased?

Instilling Helpfulness with Rewards and Models

Increasing Awareness of the Barriers to Helping

LEARNING OBJECTIVES

After reading Chapter 11, you should be able to do the following:

1. Define prosocial behaviour. Define altruism. (p. 389)

2. Identify two basic assumptions of the approach of evolutionary psychology. Discuss the three factors that explain altruism according to evolutionary theory. (pp. 390-393)

3. Describe social exchange theory. Indicate how this theory is different from sociobiological theory in its explanation of altruism. Provide examples of rewards and costs associated with helping behaviours. (pp. 393-394)

4. Describe the empathy-altruism hypothesis. Describe the debate that has arisen over whether empathy-driven helping is altruistic or egoistic. Describe research that attempts to provide evidence in support of the empathy-altruism hypothesis. (pp. 395-399)

5. Define altruistic personality. Indicate the limits to predicting helpfulness on the basis of personality and indicate what else we need to know in order to predict how helpful someone will be. (pp. 399-400)

6. Describe the effects of mood on helping. Identify why a good mood and a bad mood can result in helping behaviour. (pp. 400-402)

7. Describe the relationship between gender and forms of prosocial behaviour. Discuss reasons why males are more likely to help in some situations while females are more likely to help in others. Discuss cultural differences in prosocial behaviour. (pp. 402-404)

8. Explain why, according to the urban-overload hypothesis, people in rural environments are more helpful than people in urban environments. (pp. 405-406).

9. Describe the bystander effect. Identify and describe the step-by-step description of how people decide whether to intervene in an emergency. Describe the processes that may lead to nonintervention at each step in the decision tree. Discuss how bystanders influence pluralistic ignorance and the diffusion of responsibility and why these factors decrease helping behaviour. (pp. 406-413)

10. Describe the relationship between helping and type of relationship. Discuss the importance of rewards in an exchange versus a communal relationship. Identify when helping a friend can threaten one's self-esteem and reduce helping. (pp. 413-415)

11. Identify how helping others can make them feel. Discuss ways to increase prosocial behaviour by applying lessons learned about what increases and decreases prosocial behaviour. (pp. 416-420)

KEY TERMS

prosocial behaviour (p. 389)

altruism (p. 389)

kin selection (p. 390)

norm of reciprocity (p. 392)

empathy (p. 395)

empathy-altruism hypothesis (p. 395)

altruistic personality (p. 399)

negative-state relief hypothesis (p. 402)

in-group (p. 404)

out-group (p. 404)

urban-overload hypothesis (p. 405)

bystander effect (p. 408)

pluralistic ignorance (p. 410)

diffusion of responsibility (p. 411)

STUDY QUESTIONS

1. What is the difference between prosocial behaviour and altruism?

   —act performed benefitting another person vs. desire to help another regardless of cost to helper. (eg. harm).

2. How does the theory of evolutionary psychology explain altruism?
- for furthese survival: thru kin selection, helping a genetic relative; thru norm of reciprocity, expectation that helping others will increase the likelihood of future help from the recipient; learning social norms = adaptive.

3. What is the basic assumption of social exchange theory as it relates to prosocial behaviour? How is social exchange theory's explanation different from the evolutionary one? How is helping others rewarding? How is helping others costly?
- what we do stems from the desire to maximize rewards & minimize costs to ours.
- will help when in best interest to do so, but not when costs outweigh benefits.
⇒ disturbance c seeing another suffer ⇒ helps to alleviate own distress (rewarding).
⇒ physical danger, pain, embarassment

4. How does the empathy-altruism hypothesis explain altruistic behaviour? What are experimental strategies used to test the strength of this hypothesis? What other motives besides empathy could lead to helping?
- when we feel empathy for another, will help regardless of gains/costs.
- w/low empathy, social exchange concerns, base decision to help on costs/benefits to self (eg. sharing class notes).
- sometimes construe helping in exchange terms, to protect self from constant helping.

5. What are three basic motives that could explain prosocial behaviour?
- instinctive reaction to protect those genetically similar to us (evolutionary)
- when rewards outweigh costs, self-interest (social exchange theory)
- feelings of empathy/compassion prompt selfless giving (empathy-altruism hypothesis).

6. What is the altruistic personality? How can this personality be developed? How should rewards be used to encourage prosocial behaviour in children?
- aspects of a person's personality causing them to offer help across situations.
- develop thru rewards, comment on being "kind, helpful people", model behaviour.
- do not emph. rewards too strongly.

7. Why is knowing a person's personality not enough information to predict whether this person will engage in prosocial behaviour? What other factors are important for predicting prosocial behaviour?
- need to consider situation; prosocial behaviour not correlated w/other prosocial behav.
⇒ transitory emotional states: good/bad mood, gender, cultural diffs.

8. How do males and females differ in the area of prosocial behaviour?
- males help in brief, chivalrous acts of heroism
- women help in long-term nurturing capacities that require commitment.

9. What are cultural differences in prosocial behaviour?
- people of interdependent cultures less likely to help members of an out-group
(some) - interdependent cultures do not seek recognition for behaviour.

10. When and why do people in a good mood help others?
- b/c see others more positively
- to prolong good mood
- to increase self-estm → likely to behave according to values & ideals.

11. What is the negative-state relief hypothesis and what does it attempt to explain?

- people help others to alleviate own distress & sadness, to make selves feel better.

12. What aspects of the social situation are important for prosocial behaviour to occur? What is the relationship between population size and prosocial behaviour? How does the urban-overload hypothesis explain the greater likelihood of prosocial behaviour in towns of certain population sizes?

- rural environment, people more likely to help.
- w/ greater density of people, less likely to help; as per urban-overload hypothesis, people keep to themselves in urban areas to avoid overstimulation.

13. What are the five steps that depict what people consider when deciding whether to intervene in an emergency? What influences whether people will continue through the steps and eventually help?

1) Notice the Event
2) Interpret the Event as Emergency (beware of "pluralistic ignorance").
3) Assume Responsibility (beware of "diffusion of responsibility")
4) Knowing How to Help
5) Deciding to Implement the Help.

14. Why does the presence of other people influence people's interpretation of an event as an emergency? How does informational social influence lead to the bystander effect? What are the consequences of the bystander effect?

- "pluralistic ignorance" - people rely on others for info (informational social infl.) & assume nothing wrong if others look unconcerned.
- as a consequence, people do not believe emergency & ignore.

15. How do motives to help differ in exchange versus communal relationships?

- people concerned w/ how much each person gets in exchange r'ships
- people less concerned w/ personal benefits, more concerned w/ needs of other person in communal r'ships.

16. What are strategies to increase prosocial behaviour? What factors are important to consider when attempting to make prosocial behaviour more common?

- reward (not overcy), praise, statements of being "kind, helpful people, model prosocial behaviour, awareness of barriers to helping.

PRACTICE QUIZ CHAPTER 11

Fill-in-the-Blank

1. Any act that is performed with the goal of benefiting another person is called
_____.

2. Helping another with no thoughts about oneself is called _____.

3. The notion that behaviours which help a genetic relative are favoured by natural selection is called _____.

4. The assumption that others will treat us the way we treat them is called the
_____.

5. The theory that attempts to explain social behaviour by stressing the contributions of genetic factors and the principles of natural selection is called _____ psychology.

6. The ability to experience the events and emotions that another person is experiencing is called _____.

7. We will attempt to help a person regardless of what we have to gain if we feel empathy for that person. This is the rationale of the _____.

8. Those aspects of a person's make-up which are said to make him or her likely to help others in a wide variety of situations comprise a(n) _____.

9. The group with which one identifies and feels a sense of membership is called a(n)
_____.

10. The hypothesis that states people help others in order to alleviate their own sadness and distress is called the _____.

11. The hypothesis that maintains city dwellers keep to themselves in order to avoid excessive stimulation is called the _____.

12. The greater number of bystanders who witness an emergency, the less likely anyone is to help. This finding has been termed the _____.

13. A phenomenon whereby everyone assumes that nothing is wrong in an emergency because no one else looks concerned is called _____.

14. A decrease in the obligation people feel to help someone as the number of other witnesses increases is called _____.

Multiple Choice

15. Prosocial behaviour is
a) performed without any regard to self-interests.
b) appreciated by everyone we help.
c) performed with the goal of benefiting another person.
d) all of the above

16. The notion of kin selection dictates that you are most likely to help someone who is
a) genetically similar to you.
b) a potential mate.
c) physically attractive.
d) likely to return the favour.

17. According to social exchange theory, relationships are best understood by
    a)   assuming that others will treat us the way we treat them.
    b)   realising that people desire to maximise their benefits and minimise their costs.
    c)   applying evolutionary theory to social behaviour.
    d)   examining people's use of information gleaned by observing others in the situation.

18. Batson's empathy-altruism hypotheses states that we will help a victim of misfortune regardless of whether helping is in our best interests if
    a)   we perceive that the victim is dissimilar to us.
    b)   the costs of helping are minimal.
    c)   the victim is unable to control his or her performance.
    d)   we experience the victim's pain and suffering.

19. Maria is more likely than John to help a(n)
    a)   child in a burning building.
    b)   pilot struggling from the wreckage of an airplane.
    c)   man drowning in a lake.
    d)   elderly neighbour do his weekly shopping.

20. People in interdependent cultures are _____ likely to help members of the _____ than are people in individualistic cultures.
    a)   less; in group
    b)   more; out group
    c)   less; out group
    d)   there are no cultural differences in prosocial behaviour

21. Which of the following best characterizes the effects of mood on helping behaviour?
    a)   Good moods increase helping.
    b)   Bad moods increase helping.
    c)   Either good or bad moods can increase helping.
    d)   Neither good nor bad moods can increase helping.

22. According to Cialdini's negative-state relief hypotheses, people help others in order to
    a)   alleviate the sadness and distress of others.
    b)   alleviate their own sadness and distress.
    c)   prolong the good mood they're in.
    d)   reap the rewards of favours reciprocated in the future.

23. The Bystander Effect can be defined as
    a)   the attempt to help people regardless of what we have to gain.
    b)   the likelihood that any one person will help decreases as the number of witnesses to an emergency increases.
    c)   the assumption that others will treat us the way we treat them.
    d)   the likelihood that people will perform impulsive and deviant acts increases as group size increases.

24. Having identified a situation as a clear emergency requiring help, helping may still be inhibited by _____.
    a) pluralistic ignorance
    b) diffusion of responsibility
    c) distraction
    d) overjustification

25. Having read the chapter on prosocial behaviour, you may be more likely to offer others help because
    a) you realise that people often need help to accomplish a task even when receiving help threatens their self-esteem.
    b) you are now aware that the norm of reciprocity is universally accepted.
    c) being aware of the barriers to helping can increase the likelihood that people can overcome these barriers.
    d) viewing social exchanges as business exchanges makes it easier to recognise when helping is mutually beneficial to both you and a victim.

26. Which of the following concepts have evolutionary psychologists used to explain prosocial behaviour?
    a) kin selection and norms of reciprocity
    b) empathy and altruism
    c) immediate rewards and punishments
    d) urban overload and diffusion of responsibility

27. Parents who want to their children to grow up to exhibit prosocial behaviour should
    a) tell their children that their prosocial behaviour results from their kind and helpful nature.
    b) emphasise to their children that instances of prosocial behaviour will be rewarded.
    c) punish their children for failing to exhibit prosocial behaviours.
    d) all of the above

28. Why do researchers typically find that people who score high on personality tests of altruism are no more likely to help than those who score low?
    a) Because personality tests of altruism are invalid.
    b) Because situational influences also determine helping behaviour.
    c) Because people's personalities change greatly over time.
    d) Because altruism can be instilled in children who might otherwise not score high on personality tests of altruism.

29. People experiencing guilt tend to be helpful because
    a) they often act on the idea that good deeds cancel out bad deeds.
    b) they are more likely to interpret situations as emergencies.
    c) they are more likely to notice situations in which emergencies occur.
    d) gratitude from the victim will reassure them that they are still likeable.

30. Milgram's (1970) urban-overload hypothesis states that people in cities are less likely to help than people in rural areas because city dwellers
   a) are more aware of the negative consequences of helping.
   b) are less likely to know what form of assistance they should give.
   c) keep to themselves in order to avoid excess stimulation.
   d) are more likely to use confused bystanders as a source of misinformation.

31. Latane and Darley (1970) attributed the murder of Kitty Genovese to the
   a) large number of bystanders who witnessed the emergency.
   b) small number of bystanders who witnessed the emergency.
   c) lessons that city dwellers learn about keeping to themselves.
   d) insufficient amount of stimulation experienced by the witnesses.

32. In which type of relationship are people concerned less with equity and more with how much help is needed by the other person?
   a) exchange relationships
   b) social relationships
   c) romantic relationships
   d) communal relationships

33. Which of the following best illustrates the kind of thinking influenced by diffusion of responsibility throughout a group?
   a) "Everyone seems to be reacting calmly. Maybe there's no real problem."
   b) "I hope I don't make things worse than they already are by trying to help."
   c) "Why should I risk helping when others could as easily help?"
   d) "If no one else is offering help, I guess it's up to me."

Short Essay

34. At a concert you see a person lying on the ground moaning and assume that this person is ill. Even though you are not a doctor, you decide to go and help this person. Describe this prosocial act from the perspective of social exchange theory.

35. Distinguish between prosocial and altruistic behaviour. Why is it difficult for researchers to determine whether people ever help for purely altruistic reasons?

36. Having just slipped on a busy sidewalk, you feel a searing pain in your leg and fear that it is broken. Because you are familiar with Latane and Darley's bystander intervention decision tree, you realise that people may not help for a variety of reasons. What might you do to facilitate people's decision to help you at each stage in the decision tree?

37. By considering the situational determinants of prosocial behaviour, describe the steps you can take to increase helping among others.

38. Describe the basic motives underlying prosocial behaviour according to the evolutionary approach, social exchange theory, and the empathy-altruism hypothesis.

39. Imagine that you have just taken a drug which, your doctor tells you, has the side effect of prolonging whatever mood you are in. This, unfortunately, is bad news because you are presently experiencing some sadness and distress. As you leave the doctor's office, a man falls down in front of you. How does the negative-state relief hypothesis predict you will behave and why?

CHAPTER 12

Aggression: Why We Hurt Other People

CHAPTER OVERVIEW

Aggression is a complicated concept that is defined and elaborated upon in the first section of this chapter. The study of human aggression has led philosophers and scientists to wonder about basic human nature. A common question is concerned with the degree to which aggression is innate or learned. To help answer this question, cross-cultural research findings are discussed.

The next section focuses on the situational and biological causes of aggression. The contributing factors of the brain and hormones, alcohol, pain and discomfort, and viewing media violence in the exhibition of aggressive behaviour are examined. Situations that cause us pain, discomfort, or frustration facilitate aggression. Since aggression is largely a learned response that is more likely to be made after observing aggressive models, television violence and violent pornography have been found to be related to increases in aggression.

In the final section, strategies we might use to reduce aggressive behaviour are reviewed. Aggression can be reduced by punishment only under certain conditions. These situations are outlined. Although intuitively appealing, the catharsis hypothesis, which states that venting anger reduces future aggressive tendencies, has not been validated in research. Other options to deal with aggressive feelings and reduce another's aggression are proposed.

CHAPTER OUTLINE

What Is Aggression?

      Is Aggression Inborn, or Is It Learned?

      Is Aggression Instinctual? Situational? Optional?

      Aggressiveness Across Cultures

Neural and Chemical Causes of Aggression

      Testosterone

      Alcohol

Situational Causes of Aggression

      Pain and Discomfort as a Cause of Aggression

      Frustration as a Cause of Aggression

Direct Provocation and Reciprocation

Social Exclusion

Aggressive Objects as a Cause of Aggression

Imitation and Aggression

The Effects of Watching Media Violence

Violent Pornography and Sexual Aggression

How to Reduce Aggression

Does Punishing Aggression Reduce Aggressive Behaviour?

Catharsis and Aggression

What Are We Supposed to Do with Our Anger?

LEARNING OBJECTIVES

After reading Chapter 12, you should be able to do the following:

1. Identify the critical feature that distinguishes aggressive from nonaggressive behaviour. Explain why behaviour that causes no physical harm to anyone can still be considered aggressive behaviour. Distinguish between hostile and instrumental aggression. (pp. 425-426)

2. Contrast the philosophy of Rousseau with the philosophies of Hobbes and Freud concerning people's natural inclinations to aggress. Define Freud's concepts of Eros and Thanatos, and describe his hydraulic theory. (p. 426)

3. Discuss animal studies which support the role of instinct and those which support the role of learning in the production of aggressive behaviour. Discuss support for the learning explanation from findings that indicate innate patterns of human behaviour are infinitely modifiable and flexible. (pp. 426-427)

4. Identify the importance of culture and social change in the degree of human aggression that exists. (pp. 427-429)

5. Identify the relationship between the body and aggressive responses. Describe conditions when stimulation of the amygdala produces aggression and when it produces escape behaviour. Describe evidence that suggests the male sex hormone, testosterone, produces aggression. Discuss the relationship between gender, culture, and aggressive behaviour. Discuss the relationship between alcohol use and aggression. (pp. 429-433)

6.   Describe anecdotal and experimental evidence that suggests people are more likely to behave aggressively when they experience pain or discomfort. Identify the environmental factor that has been linked to riots and violent crime. (pp. 433-435)

7.   Describe the frustration-aggression theory. Identify factors that accentuate frustration and thereby increase the probability of aggressive behaviour. Discuss the mediating role of anger or annoyance in the frustration-aggression theory. Identify situational factors that might exacerbate aggression by someone who is frustrated. Define relative deprivation and discuss its impact on frustration and subsequent aggression. (pp. 435-437)

8.   Identify conditions when direct provocation and social exclusion are likely to evoke aggressive retaliation. (pp. 437-439)

9.   Discuss the cognitive and behavioural effects of aggressive stimuli (e.g., guns) in the presence of angry individuals. Discuss evidence that the presence of guns increases the aggressive behaviour of people in the real world. (pp. 439-441)

10.   Describe social learning theory and the basic procedure used by Bandura and his colleagues to demonstrate social learning in the laboratory. Discuss the consequences of exposing children to an aggressive model. (pp. 441-442)

11.   Discuss the effects of watching violence in the media. Identify the conclusions that can be drawn from correlational and experimental research on media violence and aggressive behaviour in children and adults. Describe evidence that suggests repeated exposure to TV violence has a numbing effect. Identify four reasons why media violence produces aggression. (pp. 442-448)

12.   Discuss the effects of viewing pornographic material on the acceptance of sexual violence toward women and on aggressive behaviour toward them. (pp. 448-450)

13.   Identify the conditions under which punishing aggression reduces aggressive behaviour in children and adults. (pp. 450-454)

14.   Define catharsis. Describe evidence that "blowing off steam" by engaging in physical activities, by watching others engage in aggressive behaviour, or by behaving aggressively increases rather than decreases hostile feelings. (pp. 454-458)

15.   Identify the most effective means of dealing with pent-up anger. Identify the benefits and underlying process of expressing feelings in a nonviolent manner. Identify an apology as an effective means of defusing anger that someone is experiencing as a consequence of your behaviour. (pp. 458-461)

16.   Discuss the effects of training, reinforcing, and of modelling nonaggressive behaviours on aggression in children. Discuss the effects of empathy and empathy training on reducing aggression. (pp. 461-462)

KEY TERMS

aggression (p. 425)

hostile aggression (p. 425)

instrumental aggression (p. 425)

Eros (p. 426)

Thanatos (p. 426)

amygdala (p. 429)

testosterone (p. 429)

frustration-aggression theory (p. 435)

relative deprivation (p. 436)

aggressive stimulus (p. 439)

social learning theory (p. 441)

catharsis (p. 454)

empathy (p. 462)

STUDY QUESTIONS

1. What is an aggression? Why is aggression difficult to define?

2. What is the difference between hostile and instrumental aggression?

3. How do Freud's Eros, Thanatos, and hydraulic theory explain human aggression?

4. What factors besides instinct determine if an animal will behave aggressively?

5.   What are cultural and regional differences in human aggressive behaviour that have been documented throughout history? What do these findings tell us about the importance of instinct in driving human aggression?

6.   What roles do the amygdala and testosterone play in aggressive behaviour? What research findings support the influence of testosterone on aggressive behaviour?

7.   Under what conditions is the consumption of alcohol related to aggressive behaviour?

8.   How are pain and heat related to aggressive behaviour?

9.   How does the frustration-aggression theory explain aggressive behaviour? What situations produce frustration? Why is relative deprivation more likely to lead to frustration and aggression than simply deprivation?

10.   How do aggressive stimuli increase the probability of aggressive behaviour? What are data that support the relationship between aggressive stimuli and aggressive behaviour?

11.   How does social learning theory explain aggressive behaviour? What is evidence that supports the explanations provided by this theory?

12.   What are the effects of watching media violence on children and adults? What are the effects of constant exposure to media violence? Why might media violence increase aggressive behaviour?

13. What are the consequences of viewing violent pornography on aggressive behaviour in general and toward women in particular?

14. What type of punishment is most likely to deter aggressiveness? Why is the threat of punishment not always an effective deterrent?

15. What are the assumptions of the catharsis hypothesis? Does engaging in aggressive or physical behaviour reduce future aggressive behaviour? What are the cognitive implications of behaving aggressively toward another? How does acting aggressively toward someone affect one's feelings toward this individual? How does cognitive dissonance theory explain these findings?

16. What effects does wartime have on a nation's aggressive behaviour at home and on attitudes toward victims abroad?

17. What are other possible strategies to reduce aggressive tendencies besides venting them? Why does "opening up" reduce aggression? How can individuals who cause frustration reduce aggression in those they have frustrated?

18. How effective are modelling and communication training at reducing aggression? What can empathy do to aggressive tendencies and the ill treatment of victims?

PRACTICE QUIZ CHAPTER 12

Fill-in-the-Blank

1. Internal behaviour aimed at causing either physical or psychological pain is called _____.

2. An act of aggression stemming from feelings of anger and aimed at inflicting pain is called _____.

3. Aggression as a means to some goal other than causing pain is called _____.

4. The instinct toward life that Freud theorised all humans are born with is called _____.

5. The instinctual drive toward death that Freud said leads to aggressive actions is called _____.

6. An area in the core of the brain that is associated with aggressive behaviour is called the _____.

7. A hormone associated with aggression is called _____.

8. The theory that frustration will increase the probability of an aggressive response is called _____.

9. The perception that you (or your group) have less than what you deserve, what you have been led to expect, or what people similar to you have, is known as _____.

10. An object that is associated with aggressive responses and whose mere presence can increase the probability of aggression is called a(n) _____.

11. The theory that people learn social behaviour by observing others and imitating them is called _____.

12. The notion that "blowing off steam" relieves built up aggressive energies and hence reduces the likelihood of further aggressive behaviour is called _____.

Multiple Choice

13. Which of the following behaviours best demonstrates instrumental aggression?
    a) shooting clay pigeons with a shotgun
    b) intentionally tripping a classmate during recess
    c) running a stop sign, thereby causing an accident
    d) holding up a clerk while robbing a convenience store

14. There is much evidence to support the general contention held by most social psychologists that, for humans, innate patterns of behaviour are
    a) rigidly preprogrammed.
    b) nonexistent.
    c) infinitely modifiable and flexible.
    d) incompatible with a social existence.

15. Research reveals that naturally occurring testosterone levels are higher among prisoners
    a) with neurological disorders.
    b) convicted of violent crimes.
    c) with personality disorders.
    d) convicted of embezzlement.

16. Carlsmith and Anderson (1979) found that riots between 1967 and 1971 were far more likely to occur on
    a)   hot days than on cool days.
    b)   rainy days than on sunny days.
    c)   weekends than on weekdays.
    d)   odd-numbered years than on even-numbered years.

17. Findings by Berkowitz and LePage (1967) that angry participants were more likely to deliver shocks to a fellow student when a gun was present in the room indicate that
    a)   the presence of weapons increases the probability that frustration will occur.
    b)   the presence of weapons in and of itself is sufficient to trigger aggressive actions.
    c)   the presence of weapons increases the probability an aggressive response will occur.
    d)   all of the above

18. At recess, a boy can choose to play with one of four classmates. Which classmate should he AVOID if he wants to play a nonviolent game of basketball?
    a)   Johnny, who tends to be aggressive and has just watched Mr. Rogers on television.
    b)   Rich, who is generally not aggressive and has just watched a violent cartoon on television.
    c)   Sam, who tends to be aggressive and has just watched a violent cartoon on television.
    d)   Tim, who is generally not aggressive and has just watched Mr. Rogers on television.

19. Physical punishment may not curb aggressive actions by children because such punishment
    a)   is difficult for children to understand.
    b)   is not supported by social norms.
    c)   models aggressive behaviour.
    d)   provides insufficient justification for behaving nonaggressively.

20. Research shows that "blowing off steam" by engaging in competitive and aggressive games or by watching others do so
    a)   increases aggressive feelings.
    b)   decreases aggressive feelings.
    c)   evokes people's primary tendencies.
    d)   inhibits aggressive behaviour.

21. Dissonance arises when we aggress toward someone who is deserving of our retaliation because
    a)   our retaliations are often more hurtful than the act for which we are retaliating.
    b)   we often fail to perceive that people are deserving of retaliation.
    c)   we often underestimate the impact retaliation has on deserving victims.
    d)   we do not like to think of ourselves as aggressive even when aggression is warranted.

22. If you are feeling angry with someone, what is the most effective way to deal with your anger?
    a)   Keep your feelings to yourself.
    b)   Express your anger in an aggressive manner.
    c)   Observe violence among others.
    d)   Calmly indicate that you are feeling angry and explain why.

23. Ohbuchi et al. (1989) found that participants liked a blundering experimental assistant better and were less likely to aggress toward him if
    a)   the experimenter insisted that the blunder had caused no harm.
    b)   the assistant blamed his blunder on the experimenter.
    c)   the assistant apologised for his blunder.
    d)   the assistant allowed the participants to be in the experiment a second time.

24. According to Freud, "Thanatos" is the
    a)   life instinct that humans are born with.
    b)   death instinct that drives aggressive actions.
    c)   process by which memories are pushed into the unconscious.
    d)   subconscious reenactment of the human evolutionary process.

25. Kuo's (1961) finding that a cat raised with a rat from birth refrained from attacking the rat or other rats suggests that
    a)   instincts may be inhibited by experience.
    b)   aggressive behaviour is not instinctive.
    c)   raising different species of animals together lowers the animals' levels of testosterone.
    d)   frustration is necessary to produce an aggressive response.

26. When the amygdala of a less-dominant monkey is stimulated in the presence of dominant monkeys, the less-dominant monkey exhibits
    a)   attack behaviour.
    b)   escape/avoidance behaviour.
    c)   no noticeable change in behaviour.
    d)   confusion and inconsistent behaviour.

27. The theory that predicts you will act with the intention to hurt others when you are thwarted from attaining a goal is called
a) social learning theory.
b) cathartic aggression theory.
c) frustration-aggression theory.
d) deprivation theory.

28. When the Iron Curtain in Eastern Europe crumbled, people expected the quality of their lives to dramatically improve. When economic reforms stalled, aggressive behaviour resulted from
a) deprivation.
b) social learning.
c) dehumanization.
d) relative deprivation.

29. Findings that children were more likely to beat up a Bobo doll after watching an adult do so led Bandura (1961, 1963) to conclude that
a) aggression may be learned by imitating aggressive models.
b) there are striking differences in instinctive aggressive drives among children.
c) watching aggressive behaviour is intrinsically rewarding.
d) observing aggression by adults unleashes children's inherent aggressiveness.

30. Which of the following best summarises the effects of viewing sexually explicit material on aggression toward women?
a) Viewing sexually explicit material, in and of itself, increases the likelihood of aggressive behaviour toward women.
b) Viewing materials that combine sex with violence increases the likelihood of aggressive behaviour toward women.
c) Viewing materials that combine sex with violence appears to be harmless.
d) Viewing nonviolent material that depict women as objects increases the likelihood of aggression toward women.

31. Pennebaker (1990) suggests that the beneficial effects of "opening" up and talking about one's feelings are the result of
a) blowing off steam.
b) increased insight and self-awareness.
c) revealing one's dependency on others.
d) increased empathy with others.

32. Evidence that people find it easier to aggress toward those they have dehumanised suggests that people will find it difficult to aggress toward people who
a) they feel empathy toward.
b) are dissimilar to them.
c) have not provoked them.
d) model aggressive behaviour.

Short Essay

33.   What evidence suggests that, among humans, innate patterns of aggression are modified by the surrounding culture?

34.   Imagine that you are on a debate team opposing a team from the National Rifle Association that maintains that "Gun's don't kill, people do." Based on what you know about the effects of "aggressive stimuli," defend your position that guns do kill people.

35.   What are the effects on children and adults of long-term exposure to television violence?

36.   Describe the frustration-aggression theory. What produces frustration? What is the role played by anger in this theory? According to this theory, what factors determine the likelihood that aggression will result from frustration?

37.   Outline steps you can take to reduce aggressive behaviour in yourself and others.

CHAPTER 13

Prejudice: Causes and Cures

CHAPTER OVERVIEW

The causes of and the remedies for the worldwide social phenomenon of prejudice are the focus of this chapter. The ubiquitous nature of prejudice is described in the first section. The definitions of prejudice, stereotyping, and discrimination are given. Distinctions between the emotional, cognitive, and behavioural components of prejudice are made.

The causes of prejudice are detailed next. The way we think about and categorise the world is one cause of prejudice that is examined. How stereotypes become activated and possibly revised are topics discussed. How we explain people's behaviour has also been linked to prejudice. People may make dispositional attributions about an entire group, thus perpetuating stereotypes, prejudice, and discrimination. The consequences related to such attribution formation, blaming the victim and the self-fulfilling prophecy, are explored. The allocation of resources and the competition that may result has been shown to cause prejudice, as well. The role of normative social influence is another cause of prejudice that is considered. Individual differences in prejudice are explored. These individual differences include just world beliefs, right-wing authoritarianism, religious fundamentalism and social dominance orientation. The effects of stereotyping prejudice and discrimination are evaluated. These include self-fulfilling prophecies, stereotype threats, and self-blaming attributions for discrimination.

Finally, strategies for reducing prejudice are described. Intergroup contact has been shown to reduce prejudice in certain situations. Lessons learned about the conditions necessary to make contact effective at reducing prejudice are outlined. These conditions have been used among school children via the use of jigsaw classrooms. The extended contact hypothesis is also explored.

CHAPTER OUTLINE

Prejudice: The Ubiquitous Social Phenomenon

Prejudice, Stereotyping, and Discrimination Defined

      Prejudice: The Affective Component

      Stereotypes: The Cognitive Component

      Discrimination: The Behavioural Component

What Causes Prejudice?

      The Way We Think: Social Cognition

      What We Believe: Stereotypes

      The Way We Feel: Affect and Mood

The Way We Assign Meaning: Attributional Biases

The Way We Allocate Resources: Realistic Conflict Theory

The Way We Conform: Normative Rules

Individual Differences in Prejudice

Just World Beliefs

Right-Wing Authoritarianism

Religious Fundamentalism

Social Dominance Orientation

Effects of Stereotyping, Prejudice, and Discrimination

Self-fulfilling Prophecies

Stereotype Threat

Self-Blaming Attributions for Discrimination

How Can Prejudice and Discrimination Be Reduced?

Learning Not to Hate

Revising Stereotypical Beliefs

The Contact Hypothesis

Cooperation and Interdependence: The Jigsaw Classroom

The Extended Contact Hypothesis

LEARNING OBJECTIVES

After reading Chapter 13, you should be able to do the following:

1. Describe the ubiquitous nature of prejudice. Identify what aspects of people's identities that are targeted for prejudice. Discuss the consequences of prejudice for the targets of prejudice. Describe the nature of prejudice today. (pp. 468-471)

2. Define prejudice. Describe the affective component of prejudice, the cognitive compoment, and the behavioural component. (pp. 471-475)

3. Describe the social cognition approach to the study of the causes of prejudice. Identify how schemas contribute to the social cognition approach. Why are such schemas so resistant to change? Describe social categorization and the motives underlying in-group bias. How is out-group homogeneity another consequence of social categorization? (pp. 475-482)

4. Describe the complex relationship between stereotyping and prejudice. Describe the role of automatic processes in the activation of stereotypes and of controlled processes in stereotype activation and inhibition. Explain the role of meta-stereotypes. (pp. 482-488)

5. Discuss how affect and mood can serve as a predictor of prejudice. Explain how the situation can mediate the role of emotion in predicting attitudes. (pp. 488-491)

6. Define the ultimate attribution error and discuss the influence of stereotyping in the committing of this error. (pp. 491-492)

7. Describe realistic conflict theory as well as correlational and experimental support for this theory. Discuss the relationship between economic and political competition and prejudice. (pp. 492-495)

8. Describe how stereotypes and prejudiced attitudes are sometimes the results of normative rules. Explain the term modern prejudice. Identify techniques used by researchers to reveal subtle forms of prejudice. (pp. 495-499)

9. Describe important individual differences in prejudice. Explain how the belief in a just world leads us to "blame the victim" for his or her misfortune. Define and distinguish right-wing authoritarianism, religious fundamentalism and social dominance orientation. (pp. 499-502)

10. Describe the relevance of the self-fulfilling prophecy to stereotyping and discrimination at the individual and societal levels. (pp. 502-504)

11. Discuss stereotype threat and the self-blaming by victims of discrimination (pp. 504-508)

12. Discuss learning not to hate using Jane Elliot's classroom demonstration (pp. 508-510).

13. Identify the kinds of disconfirming information necessary to result in stereotype revision by "bookkeeping," "subtyping," and "conversion". (pp. 510-511)

14. Define the contact hypothesis as stated by Allport (1954) and identify the six conditions necessary to reduce prejudice when there is contact between groups. (pp. 511-513)

15. Describe how contact between students in the jigsaw classroom differs from contact in traditional classroom settings. Identify the advantages that have been gained by students learning in jigsaw classrooms. (pp. 513-515)

16. Describe the extended contact hypothesis. (pp. 515-517)

KEY TERMS

prejudice (p. 471)

stereotype (p. 472)

discrimination (p. 473)

out-group homogeneity (p. 481)

meta-stereotype (p. 487)

ultimate attribution error (p. 491)

realistic conflict theory (p. 492)

normative conformity (p. 496)

modern prejudice (p. 496)

self-fulfilling prophecy (p. 503)

stereotype threat (p. 504)

bookkeeping model (p. 510)

conversion model (p. 510)

subtyping model (p. 510)

mutual interdependence (p. 512)

jigsaw classroom (p. 514)

extended contact hypothesis (p. 516)

STUDY QUESTIONS

1.   What are the consequences of prejudice?

2.   How is prejudice different from discrimination? What are the three components of a prejudiced attitude?

3.   How do gender stereotypes affect achievement attributions of men's and women's successes and failures? What type of attributions are made by individuals and society for the successes of men compared to those of women?

4.   What is an example of discrimination?

5.   What role does human thinking have in the causes of prejudice? How does social categorization increase prejudice? What are motives behind the in-group bias?

6.   What is the out-group homogeneity effect and how does it contribute to prejudice?

7.   What does Devine's (1989) two-step model of cognitive processing explain about prejudice?

8.   What are the characteristics of Altemeyer's authoritarian personality?

9.   What is the ultimate attribution error? What are the consequences of committing this error?

10.   What is stereotype threat and what does it help to explain?

11.   What is the relationship between the belief in a just world and blaming the victim?

12.   How does the self-fulfilling prophecy perpetuate prejudice and discrimination?

13.   According to the realistic conflict theory, what are the causes of prejudice and discrimination?

14.   How is the expression of racism and sexism in today's society different from its expression fifty years ago? How have research techniques adapted to study this "new" racism and sexism?

15.   What are effective strategies to reduce prejudice? What characteristic of intergroup contact are necessary for the contact hypothesis to reduce prejudice and discrimination? What is mutual interdependence?

16.   What are the characteristics of the jigsaw classroom? What are the benefits of the jigsaw classroom?

17.   What is the extended contact hypothesis?

PRACTICE QUIZ CHAPTER 13

Fill-in-the-Blank

1.   A hostile or negative attitude toward a distinguishable group of people, based solely on their membership in that group is called _____.

2.   A generalization about a group of people in which identical characteristics are assigned to virtually all members of the group, regardless of the actual variation among the members is called a(n) _____.

3.   The unjustified negative or harmful action toward a member of a group, simply because of his or her membership in that group, is called _____.

4.   The perception that members of the out-group are more similar to one another than they really are, and more similar to one another than are the members of one's in-group, is called the perception of _____.

5. A model for modifying stereotypic beliefs when information inconsistent with the stereotype is encountered among many members of the categorised group is called the _____ model.

6. A model for radically changing stereotypic beliefs when confronted with a fact that very strongly disconfirms the stereotype is called the _____ model.

7. A model for creating a subcategory of a stereotype when information inconsistent with the stereotype is concentrated among only a few individuals in the categorised group is called the _____ model.

8. The tendency to make dispositional attributions about an entire group of people is called the _____.

9. The theory that maintains limited resources lead to conflict between groups and result in increased prejudice and discrimination is called _____.

10. The tendency to go along with the group in order to fulfil members' expectations and gain their acceptance is called _____.

11. When two or more groups need each other and must depend on each other in order to accomplish a goal that is important to each of them, the groups are _____.

12. A technique for structuring the classroom designed to reduce prejudice and raise the self-esteem of children by placing them in small, desegregated groups and making each child dependent on the other children for his or her group to learn the material is called the _____.

13. The fear that one might behave in a manner that confirms some stereotype about your social group is called _____.

14. The _____ suggests that prejudice may be reduced by contact of equal status between majority and minority groups.

15. _____ is the collection of beliefs held about what out-group members think about their own group.

Multiple Choice

16. Once formed, stereotypes
    a) easily change when contradictory information is encountered.
    b) develop into more elaborate and complex categories.
    c) deteriorate unless challenged by contradictory information.
    d) are resistant to change on the basis of new information.

17. According to Allport, stereotypes result
    a) as the inevitable by-product of the way we process and categorise information.
    b) from the breakdown of once normal cognitive processes.
    c) from conflicts that exist between groups when resources are limited.
    d) when individuals adhere to norms which foster prejudice.

18. According to Devine's (1989) two-step model of cognitive processing, simply knowing stereotypes that you do not believe affects your cognitive processing because
    a) we are constantly aware of the stereotypes.
    b) we can recall the stereotypes at will.
    c) the stereotypes are inconsistent with our beliefs.
    d) the stereotypes are automatically activated.

19. Realistic conflict theory maintains that
    a) abundant resources produces greed and negative feelings toward out-groups.
    b) conflict experienced within a group is likely to be attributed to members of an out-group.
    c) mutual interdependence among groups produces competition and negative feelings toward competing groups.
    d) limited resources produce competition and negative feelings toward competing groups.

20. Prejudice is
    a) any behaviour aimed at physically or emotionally harming people who are members of a discernible group.
    b) a generalization about a group of people in which identical characteristics are assigned to virtually all members of the group.
    c) a hostile or negative attitude toward a distinguishable group of people, based solely on their membership in that group.
    d) the tendency to categorise people into groups based on some specific characterisation.

21. The bigot's cry, "they all look alike to me," illustrates one consequence of social categorisation called the
    a) perception of out-group homogeneity.
    b) in-group bias.
    c) illusory correlation.
    d) ultimate attribution error.

22. Furnham and Gunter (1984) have found that negative attitudes toward the poor and homeless are more prevalent among individuals who
    a) score high on measures of self-esteem.
    b) tend to be high in self-awareness.
    c) believe we live in a "dog-eat-dog" world.
    d) have a strong belief in a "just world."

23. According to Allport (1954), contact between majority and minority groups will reduce prejudice when members of the groups
    a) interact voluntarily in an unstructured setting.
    b) have low expectations for increased intergroup harmony.
    c) compete for limited available resources.
    d) are of equal status and in pursuit of common goals.

24. Individuals high on _____ are most well-defined by their belief that some people are better than other people.
    a) social dominance orientation
    b) religious fundamentalism
    c) right-wing authoritarianism
    d) racial prejudice

25. Word, Zanna and Cooper found that when white university undergraduates displayed discomfort and a lack of interest while interviewing African Americans job applicants, the African Americans appeared
    a) aggressive and hostile
    b) nervous and far less effective
    c) poised, effective and competent
    d) unaffected by the behaviour of the white university undergraduates

26. A(n) _____ explanation for prejudice suggests the way we process and organize information causes prejudice.
    a) social cognition
    b) personality
    c) self-esteem
    d) economic factors

27. According to research by Gardner and colleagues, if asked to describe the stereotypical male, all the following characteristics should be rated more quickly except
    a) rugged
    b) artistic
    c) impatient
    d) talkative

28. Kyle holds negative stereotypes of natives but received very positive feedback from his employer who is native. Research by Sinclair and Kunda suggests that Kyle's reaction will be to
    a) reject the positive feedback
    b) make negative attributions about the motives of his employer
    c) set aside his negative stereotypes towards natives in this instance
    d) seek feedback from non-native others

29. According to research by Hoddock and colleagues (1993), the best predictor of attitudes toward an ethnic group is your
    a) feelings toward members of that group
    b) beliefs about members of that group
    c) perceptions of what members of the group value
    d) behaviour toward members of that group

30. The idea of _____ suggests you may display prejudiced attitudes in order to be popular with your friends.
    a) authoritarian personality
    b) normative conformity
    c) modern prejudice
    d) jigsaw classroom

31. In a study by Shih, Pittinsky and Ambady (1999), Asian-American female university students were administered the Canadian Math Competition Test. Participants who scored highest on the test did so after being reminded they were
    a) female
    b) Asian
    c) female and Asian
    d) not Canadian

32. The extended contact hypothesis suggests that prejudice can be reduced by
    a) spending time travelling
    b) attending university classes
    c) making friends with a member of another group
    d) confronting your prejudiced attitudes

Short Essay

33. Why, according to Devine's two-step model of cognitive processing, are people who are high in prejudice more likely to express stereotypic thinking than people who are low in prejudice?

34. How does the self-fulfilling prophesy serve to perpetuate biased expectations produced by the ultimate attribution error?

35. During the past couple of months, you have become increasingly aware and concerned that a friend of yours is prejudiced against a particular ethnic group on campus. Explain why you will anticipate having a difficult time eliminating your friend's prejudice by presenting evidence that disconfirms his stereotype. Propose a model for modifying stereotypic beliefs with disconfirming evidence that may work under these difficult conditions.

36. How have children in jigsaw classrooms benefited from learning in this environment?

SOCIAL PSYCHOLOGY IN ACTION 1

Social Psychology and Health

OVERVIEW

People's awareness of issues related to their health has increased tremendously in the past decade. Research has revealed that our physical health is affected by our interpretation of events as stressful, by the amount of control we feel over such events, and by the way we explain negative outcomes. The way in which we cope with stress is also important for our health. The module discusses two main personality types and their relationship with poor health. The effective coping styles of "opening up" and social support are also discussed. Understanding these issues from the perspective of a social psychologist suggests some ways to change behaviour that is detrimental to people's health. The final section reviews how the use of social psychological principles can improve health habits.

OUTLINE

Stress and Human Health

    Effects of Negative Life Events

    Perceived Stress and Health

    Feeling in Charge: The Importance of Perceived Control

    Knowing You Can Do It: Self-Efficacy

    Explaining Negative Events: Learned Helplessness

Coping with Stress

    Personality and Coping Styles

    "Opening Up": Confiding to Others

    Social Support: Getting Help From Others

Prevention: Improving Health Habits

    Message Framing: Stressing Gains versus Losses

    Changing Health-Relevant Behaviours Using Dissonance Theory

LEARNING OBJECTIVES

After reading Social Psychology in Action 1, you should be able to do the following:

1. Explain the connection between stress and health. Describe attempts to show this connection using the Social Readjustment Rating Scale. Highlight the importance of studying subjective rather than objective stress. Describe recent research that suggests stress lowers people's resistance to infectious disease. (pp. 522-527)

2. Describe correlational and experimental research that suggests perceived control is associated with better adjustment to chronic diseases, greater immunity to disease, and with better health and adjustment among residents of nursing homes. Distinguish between the effects of a temporary and an enduring sense of control. (pp. 528-532)

3. Define self-efficacy. Describe two ways that self-efficacy increases the likelihood that people will engage in healthier behaviours. Describe how self-efficacy can be increased. (pp. 532-533)

4. Describe the attributions for negative events that result in learned helplessness and depression. Describe the link between learned helplessness and academic performance. Discuss the association between a pessimistic attributional style and health. (pp. 534-537)

5. Discuss research on personality and coping styles. Discuss how personality can affect health. Identify the characteristics of the Type A and the Type B personalities. Identify the characteristic of a Type A that can lead health problems. Discuss how the Type A and the Type B may develop. Discuss cultural differences in the incidence of coronary disease and how this may be linked to individualism versus collectivism. Define hardiness and its relationship to stress. (pp. 537-541)

6. Discuss the effectiveness of "opening up" as a coping style. Explain why "opening up" can lead to better health. (pp. 541-542)

7. Identify the health benefits of social support. Discuss cross-cultural differences in the existence of social support and the consequences of these differences. Define the buffering hypothesis. Discuss two ways that social support can help in times of stress. (pp. 543-544)

8. Discuss how social psychological principles can be applied to improve health by reducing stress and by getting people to change their health habits. Discuss the role of message framing to stress gains rather than losses and the role of the arousal of cognitive dissonance in inducing change. (pp. 544-549)

KEY TERMS

stress (p. 524)

perceived control (p. 528)

136

self-efficacy (p. 532)

stable attribution (p. 534)

internal attribution (p. 534)

global attribution (p. 534)

learned helplessness (p. 534)

coping styles (p. 537)

Type A versus B personality (p. 538)

hardiness (p. 540)

social support (p. 543)

buffering hypothesis (p. 544)

STUDY QUESTIONS

1. What are definitions of stress? What are the Social Readjustment Rating Scale and "life change units" and their relationship to stress? What factor has been found to be important in determining what is stressful for people?

2. What are the consequences of subjective stress for one's health?

3. How important is perceived control over events in one's life for reducing the perception and detrimental effects of stress? What is learned helplessness, how does it develop, and what are its consequences?

4. What is self-efficacy? How does the perception of it affect one's health?

5. How do findings from studies conducted in nursing homes confirm the importance of perceived control for reducing stress? Why is it better to have never had control than to have had it and have had it taken away? When is the perception of control problematic for one's psychological and physical health?

6. How and why are attributions an important determinant of stress? What are the three aspects of a pessimistic attribution? What are the consequences of making pessimistic attributions?

7. How are learned helplessness, attributional style, and achievement related? What can we do to reduce learned helplessness in first-year college students? What influences the development of attributional styles?

8. What is the relationship between coping styles, personality, and health? What are the characteristics of a Type A and a Type B personality? What factors determine if people have a Type A or a Type B personality? What is the main aspect of a Type A personality that has been found to be related to health problems?

9. Why is "opening up" a successful coping style? What are the long-term benefits of "opening up" in response to a negative life event?

10. Why is the availability and use of social support a successful way to deal with stress? What benefits exist in collectivist cultures regarding the availability of social support? What does the buffering hypothesis propose regarding the necessity of social support?

11. How can we help people engage in healthy behaviours? What important social psychological techniques would be helpful in getting people to live healthier lives? What may be one of the best ways to change people's behaviour and solve applied problems?

PRACTICE QUIZ SOCIAL PSYCHOLOGY IN ACTION 1

Fill-in-the-Blank

1.   The negative feelings and beliefs that occur whenever people feel that they cannot cope with demands from their environment are called _____.

2.   The belief that we can influence our environment in ways that determine whether we experience positive or negative outcomes is called _____.

3.   The belief that one can perform a given behaviour that produces desired results is called _____.

4.   The state of pessimism that results from explaining a negative event as due to stable, internal, and global causes is called _____.

5.   The belief that the cause of an event is due to factors that will not change over time is called a(n) _____.

6.   The belief that the cause of an event is due to things about you, such as your ability or effort, is called a(n) _____.

7.   The belief that the cause of an event is due to factors that apply in a large number of situations is called a(n) _____.

8.   The ways in which people react to stressful events are called _____.

9.   A person who is typically competitive, impatient, and hostile is called a(n) _____ and a person who is typically more patient, relaxed, and noncompetitive is called a(n) _____.

10.   The perception that others are responsive and receptive to one's needs is called _____.

11.   The _____ stresses the importance of social support when we are facing the effects of negative life events.

Multiple Choice

12.   Stress is the
       a)   state of pessimism that results from attributing a negative event to stable, internal, and global causes.
       b)   inability to control the outcomes of one's efforts.
       c)   awareness of heightened physiological arousal.
       d)   negative feelings and beliefs that occur whenever people feel they cannot cope with demands from their environment.

13. Many North Americans have begun to reject aspects of the traditional medical model, especially the submissive role expected of patients by many doctors. One reason why this new approach to medicine may be catching on is that patients
    a) gain a more objective conceptualisation of health issues.
    b) benefit from greater perceived control over their illness.
    c) enjoy the status that is usually reserved for medical doctors.
    d) pay lower insurance costs when they make use of nontraditional medical approaches.

14. Langer and Rodin (1976) found that nursing home residents were happier, more active, and lived longer when
    a) they were provided with interesting movies to watch.
    b) their surroundings were beautified with plants.
    c) they were given responsibility and control over decisions.
    d) the staff made potentially stressful choices for them.

15. An individual who exaggerates the role of perceived control in alleviating physical illness runs the risk of
    a) experiencing self-blame and failure if the illness persists.
    b) experiencing stress by maintaining a perception that the course of the disease is unpredictable.
    c) making unstable, external, and specific attributions if the illness persists.
    d) all of the above

16. If Ken believes that he flunked his English test because he's lazy and lacks intelligence, he is attributing his failure to ____ causes.
    a) external, unstable, and specific
    b) internal, stable, and global
    c) external, stable, and specific
    d) internal, unstable, and global

17. Research by Aronson and colleagues found that individuals were more likely to practice safe sex when they were
    a) informed of the consequences of practising unsafe sex.
    b) induced to publicly advocate safe sex.
    c) made mindful of their own failure to practice safe sex.
    d) made aware of their own hypocrisy.

18. High positive correlations between scores on Holmes and Rahe's (1967) Social Readjustment Rating Scale and the likelihood of physical illness indicate that health problems are associated with
    a) people's interpretations of their social world.
    b) a pessimistic attributional style.
    c) learned helplessness.
    d) changes in a person's life.

19. Participants in a study by Cohen et al. (1991) who experienced low or high amounts of stress were exposed to a virus that causes the common cold. Results indicated that
    a) increasing participants' awareness of the virus made them more susceptible to catching a cold.
    b) exposure to the virus is sufficient to trigger illness, regardless of the amount of stress experienced by participants.
    c) participants who experienced high amounts of stress were more likely to catch a cold.
    d) extraneous factors such as age, weight, and gender masked the relationship between stress and immunological response.

20. The unforeseen tragic results of Schulz (1976) nursing home study suggest that institutions which strive to give their patients a sense of control should ensure that
    a) patients are not overwhelmed by responsibilities.
    b) patients will not have to relinquish that control.
    c) certain restrictions on the amount of control are enforced.
    d) decisions are made for patients who do not want control.

21. If you believe that the cause of an event is due to things about you, such as your ability or effort, you are making a(n) _____ attribution.
    a) specific
    b) internal
    c) stable
    d) global

22. Which of the following factors is the most important determinant of learned helplessness?
    a) the individual's perceptions of the causes of events
    b) the accuracy of the individual's causal attributions
    c) the actual causes of events
    d) the individual's attributions for events that did not, but could have, occurred

23. Who is most likely to suffer from stress-related diseases?
    a) Joe, who is competitive, hostile, and impatient
    b) John, who is competitive, patient, and caring
    c) James, who is easygoing, relaxed, and ambitious
    d) Jerry, who is calm, noncompetitive, and reserved

24. Which of the following are successful coping styles?
    a) "opening up"
    b) becoming hostile and confrontational
    c) engaging social support
    d) both a and c

Short Essay

25. Describe means of improving people's health that have been suggested by social psychologists.

26. Imagine that you have just become the director of a home for the elderly. Describe the conditions that you would implement at the home to make residents happier and healthier.

27. Imagine that you are a clinical psychologist and a client comes to you complaining about persistent though not severe depression. Using what you know about learned helplessness theory, suggest changes in the way your client explains events that will alleviate the melancholia.

SOCIAL PSYCHOLOGY IN ACTION 2

Social Psychology and the Environment

OVERVIEW

Our reactions to environmental stimuli (e.g., noise, crowds) are largely a consequence of how stressful we perceive them to be. This module discusses how noise, crowding and toxic environments can be stressful. The harmful effects of these environmental factors are reviewed. Social psychology offers assistance in changing environmentally damaging behaviours. However, obstacles to engaging in energy conscious behaviours are social dilemmas. How we can resolve these dilemmas is examined in this module as are the successes of social psychologists at getting people to conserve water and energy. The influences of injunctive and descriptive norms on reducing littering is discussed. Also covered are ways we can get people to recycle. Finally, two strategies to increase environmental consciousness and environmentally sound behaviours are detailed.

CHAPTER OUTLINE

The Environment as a Source of Stress

> Noise as a Source of Stress

> Crowding as a Source of Stress

> Toxic Environments as a Source of Stress

Using Social Psychology to Change Environmentally Damaging Behaviour

> Resolving Social Dilemmas

> Conserving Water

> Conserving Energy

> Reducing Litter

> Getting People to Recycle

LEARNING OBJECTIVES

After reading Social Psychology in Action 2, you should be able to do the following:

1. Identify stressors that have been eliminated and others which have been created as civilisation has progressed. (pp. 554-555)

2.	Describe the conditions under which noise is psychologically stressful. Identify the effects of uncontrollable noise on health, cognitive functioning and task performance. Discuss noise in modern urban life. (pp. 555-558)

3.	Describe the effects of crowding on animal and human behaviour. Distinguish between density and crowding and identify factors that turn density into crowding. Discuss what norms other cultures have developed to avoid crowding even in a very dense environment. Describe the relationship between crowding and our expectations. Describe the relationship between the effects of crowding and attribution. Define sensory overload and its relationship to crowding. (pp. 558-562)

4.	How are toxic environments a source of stress? (p. 562)

5.	Define a social dilemma. Describe the conflict that arises when people are confronted with social dilemmas such as wastefulness and pollution. Identify conditions that decrease selfish behaviours and foster trust in response to such dilemmas. (pp. 563-566)

6.	How has the hypocrisy technique between used by Aronson and colleagues (1992) to reduce water consumption. (pp. 566-567)

7.	Explain why most consumers have not taken steps to conserve energy even when doing so would save them a great deal of money. Discuss how social psychologists persuade homeowners to conserve energy. Identify successful strategies aimed at increasing energy conservation behaviour. (pp. 567-570)

8.	Distinguish between injunctive and descriptive norms. Describe how Cialdini and colleagues have reduced littering by reminding people of these norms. Identify how descriptive norms are most effectively communicated. Identify the limitation of using descriptive norms to communicate appropriate behaviour. (pp. 570-573)

9.	Describe the inconveniences that lead many not to recycle. Describe to approaches that social psychologists have taken to encourage recycling. (pp. 573-575)

KEY TERMS

density (p. 558)

crowding (p. 558)

sensory overload (p. 562)

injunctive norms (p. 570)

descriptive norms (p. 570)

STUDY QUESTIONS

1.   When is an environment stressful? What are relatively recent environmental stressors that our civilisation has to face?

2.   When is noise psychologically stressful? What conditions are necessary to reduce the ill effects of loud noise? What are detrimental effects of uncontrollable noise? How has environmental noise affected the performance of school children?

3.   What are findings from studies of crowding in animals and humans? What psychological effects do crowded dorms have on students? Why is crowding aversive? What factors are linked with perceptions of crowding?

4.   How are the effects of noise and crowding similar?

5.   What is sensory overload and what are its consequences?

6.   According to research, how can we resolve social dilemmas?

7.   How can we get people to stop littering? What roles do injunctive and descriptive norms play in decreasing littering? Why are injunctive norms more effective than descriptive norms?

8.   What strategies have been successful at increasing energy conservation behaviours such as recycling?

PRACTICE QUIZ SOCIAL PSYCHOLOGY IN ACTION 2

Fill-in-the-blank

1.   The number of people who occupy a given space is called _____.

2.   The subjective feeling of unpleasantness due to the presence of other people is called _____.

3.   Receiving more stimulation from the environment than we can pay attention to or process leads to _____.

4.   People's perceptions of what behaviours are approved of by others are called _____.

5.   People's perceptions of how other people are actually behaving in a given situation, regardless of what they ought to be doing, are called _____.

Multiple Choice

6.   People who go to rock concerts do not find the extremely loud noise to be stressful because
a)   many other people are also present.
b)   they chose to go to the concert.
c)   norms dictate that anxiety is inappropriate for leisure activities.
d)   they cannot pay attention to all the stimulation that is encountered.

7.   Participants who solved problems while being exposed to uncontrollable and loud noise performed more poorly on subsequent problems that were solved under quiet conditions because
a)   they had adapted to the noise and were uncomfortable in its absence.
b)   they naturally lost the ability to concentrate over time.
c)   they succumbed to learned helplessness after initially fighting the noxious effects of the noise.
d)   the tasks presented during the second session were more difficult.

8.   Paulus et al. (1981) found that at crowded prisons
a)   friendships are more likely to be formed.
b)   overall death rates increase.
c)   escapes are more common.
d)   released prisoners are less likely to return.

9.   Density turns into crowding when
a)   the presence of others lowers our feelings of control.
b)   the number of people per square foot exceed the density ratio.
c)   we are unable to determine the social structure of the situation.
d)   external stimulation becomes more than we can process.

10. Though driving affords you greater personal freedom, the pollution created by millions of drivers represents a global problem. This situation is a classic example of a problem known as a(n)
   a)   high-density situation.
   b)   paradoxical affair.
   c)   social dilemma.
   d)   attributional spiral.

11. Aronson and his students increased the energy-conserving behaviour of homeowners by
   a)   reminding people of the need to make certain repairs.
   b)   publicising problems to the neighbourhood homeowner's association.
   c)   increasing people's perceived control over making such changes.
   d)   having energy auditors present their findings in a more dramatic way.

12. People's perceptions of how others are actually behaving in a given situation, regardless of what they ought to be doing are _____ norms.
   a)   injunctive
   b)   conjunctive
   c)   descriptive
   d)   global

13. In which of the following situations is littering LEAST likely?
   a)   an immaculately clean room
   b)   a badly littered room
   c)   a badly littered room with a sign prohibiting litter
   d)   an otherwise clean room with a single piece of litter

14. Rosen and his colleagues (1962) found that, compared to people living in the civilised world, primitive Mabaans
   a)   were more susceptible to physical illness.
   b)   were more likely to exhibit psychological disorders.
   c)   had less per capita violence in their culture.
   d)   had less hypertension and obesity.

15. Though you enjoy blasting your favourite tunes on your car stereo, you find it annoying when someone pulls up to you at a stoplight with their stereo blaring. A social psychologist would attribute your different reactions to loud music to
   a)   the perceived control that you have over the volume of the music.
   b)   different tastes that people acquired for music in various subcultures.
   c)   attributional biases in explaining the behaviour of others.
   d)   tension produced by dissonant cognitions about liking music and obeying social norms.

16. Compared to children who attended quiet schools, children who attended schools in the air corridor of Los Angeles Airport
    a) had higher blood pressure.
    b) were more easily distracted.
    c) were less likely to persevere on difficult problems.
    d) all of the above

17. Students will feel crowded in a classroom if
    a) there are more than twenty people in the classroom.
    b) they feel that there are too many people in the classroom.
    c) the class is very highly structured.
    d) they receive too much stimulation in the classroom.

18. Differences in people's reactions to crowding may be explained, in part, by
    a) the attributions they make for their physiological arousal.
    b) their ability to resolve cognitive dissonance.
    c) their overall level of self-esteem.
    d) their overall level of physical fitness.

19. Orbell et al. (1988) found that participants were most likely to donate money to a community pot, and thereby benefit everyone in the group, if they
    a) were made to feel dissonance between being a nice person and being selfish.
    b) first heard a sermon about the Good Samaritan.
    c) interacted with other participants for ten minutes before having to decide whether or not to donate.
    d) all of the above interventions increased donations.

20. The difficulty of getting people to conserve water and energy and to recycle their waste goods demonstrates the difficulty of resolving
    a) attributional biases.
    b) disjunctive tasks.
    c) social dilemmas.
    d) self-serving biases.

21. You are most likely to feel social pressure to conform if you are exposed to a(n) _____ norm.
    a) injunctive
    b) descriptive
    c) peripheral
    d) elaborative

22. Which types of norms depend upon everyone's cooperation in order to be effective?
    a) injunctive norms
    b) descriptive norms
    c) nonsalient norms
    d) generosity norms

Short Essay

23. If you were a member of a local water conservation committee, how might you go about inducing community members to save water when they know that it is in their own immediate best interests to use all the water that they want?

24. At a local park, littering has become a serious problem. Describe techniques you could employ to evoke injunctive and descriptive norms against littering. Which kind of norm is most likely to be effective in the long run? Why?

25. You and other members of your community are fighting to decrease noise pollution caused by jets taking off and landing at a nearby airport. What arguments might you present to officials at the Department of Transportation in order to convince them that the noise is having detrimental effects on community members?

26. Describe conditions that have been used successfully to resolve social dilemmas.

SOCIAL PSYCHOLOGY IN ACTION 3

Social Psychology and the Law

OVERVIEW

In this module, you will see how social psychologists apply principles, which by now are familiar to you, to initiate change in our legal system and promote justice for everyone involved. The application of social psychological principles to law is detailed. Although jurors are heavily influenced by eyewitness testimony, distortions in social cognition and attribution introduce unintentional error into such testimony. When a witness purposely lies, there is an even greater likelihood that testimony will distort the opinions of jurors who, like the rest of us, are not very skilled at detecting deception. Finally, jurors can be biased by publicity before the trial, by the way they process information during the trial, and by social influences that operate while the jury deliberates. Also covered in this module is the question of why people obey laws. One theory focuses on the deterrent effect of severe penalties. The importance of people's conception of a fair legal system is addressed.

CHAPTER OUTLINE

Eyewitness Testimony

     Why Are Eyewitnesses Often Wrong?

     Judging Whether Eyewitnesses Are Mistaken

     Judging Whether Eyewitnesses Are Lying

     Can Eyewitness Testimony Be Improved?

Other Kinds of Evidence

     Expert Testimony

     Physical Evidence

     Statistical Evidence

Juries: Group Processes in Action

     Effects of Pretrial Publicity

     How Juries Process Information During the Trial

     Deliberations in the Jury Room

Why Do People Obey the Law?

     Do Severe Penalties Deter Crime?

     Procedural Justice: People's Sense of Fairness

LEARNING OBJECTIVES

After reading Social Psychology in Action 3, you should be able to do the following:

1. Discuss jurors' reliance on eyewitness testimony and their tendency to overestimate the accuracy of eyewitnesses. Identify why the accuracy of such testimony is overestimated. Describe the relationship between the juror's perception of accurate testimony and eyewitness confidence. (pp. 580-581)

2. Identify situational factors that influence acquisition. Discuss the effect of previous expectancies on the acquisition of information. Define own-race bias and discuss its significant in eyewitness testimony. (pp. 581-584)

3. Contrast the notion that memories are stored in our minds as static photographs with the notion that memories are actively reconstructed. Identify the role of misleading questions in reconstructive memory. Discuss how misleading questions alter what is stored in witnesses' memories. Define source monitoring and discuss its importance. (pp. 584-587)

4. Identify the role of retrieval in identifying a suspect from a police lineup. List the six steps that social psychologists recommend to reduce the likelihood that witnesses will mistakenly pick an innocent individual out of a lineup when that person resembles the suspect. (pp. 587-589)

5. Discuss why the confidence of a witness does not necessarily equal the accuracy of his/her testimony. Identify ways to assess the accuracy of a witness' testimony. (pp. 589-592)

6. Describe the controversy over the use of the polygraph. Discuss the results of research on the accuracy of polygraph tests. Discuss why social psychologists doubt that a foolproof method of lie detection will ever be developed. (pp. 592-595)

7. Evaluate hypnosis and the cognitive interview as techniques for improving eyewitness testimony. Discuss the recovered memory debate and evidence for recovered memories. (pp. 595-597)

8. Identify the issues around expert testimony. Why have courts in Canada moved away from expert testimony? What role does physical and statistical evidence have to play in criminal trials?   (pp. 597-600)

9. Identify ways in which pretrial publicity biases jurors' verdicts. Identify legal procedures aimed at eliminating these biases and indicate their effectiveness. (pp. 600-602)

10. Describe the strategy jurors use to process information during a trial. Identify the implications for such a strategy on how lawyers present their cases. Distinguish between story order and witness order presentations of evidence. (pp. 602-603)

11. Identify the role of group processes and social interactions in the way juries reach verdicts. Discuss the role of conformity in the process of jury deliberation. Identify the effects of forcing unanimity have on jury deliberation and outcomes. (pp. 603-605)

12. Discuss the evidence on whether or not severe penalties deter crimes. Discuss the assumptions that deterrence theory makes. (pp. 605-608)

13. Define procedural justice, and discuss its role in people's obedience to the law. Discuss the factors that determine whether or not people think a law is just. (pp. 608-610)

KEY TERMS

acquisition (p. 581)

storage (p. 581)

retrieval (p. 581)

own-race bias (p. 584)

reconstructive memory (p. 585)

source monitoring (p. 586)

polygraph (p. 593)

cognitive interview (p. 597)

recovered memory (p. 597)

deterrence theory (p. 605)

procedural justice (p. 609)

STUDY QUESTIONS

1. What can social psychologists offer to the study of the legal system?

2. Why do jurors overestimate the accuracy of eyewitness testimony?

3. What are the three stages of memory processing? What can interfere with processing at each stage of memory? What conditions are present at most crime scenes and how does this affect acquisition? How do expectancies affect the acquisition of information?

4. Why is familiarity an important factor in memory processing? What is the own-race bias? What consequences does this bias have on eyewitness testimony?

5. What are the characteristics of our memory storage? What is reconstructive memory? What has been discovered about the accuracy of our memory? What is source monitoring? What effects do misleading questions have on source monitoring? Why is incorrect source monitoring a problem for eyewitness accuracy?

6. What consequences does retrieval have for the correct identification of a suspect from a police lineup? What are the six steps to follow when conducting a police lineup? What is the rationale behind each step?

7. How can we tell if a witness's testimony is accurate? Why is confidence of one's testimony not always a good estimate of the accuracy of one's testimony? What are the consequences of trying to put a face into words for the accuracy of identifying the face?

8. How well can people detect deception? Do those working in the field of law enforcement do better than others at detecting deception?

9. What is a polygraph machine designed to do and how does it do it? What is the assumption behind the use of the polygraph? How accurate, on average, are polygraphs at detecting when someone is lying? Does failing a polygraph test always mean that one is lying? Why is a machine intended to tell if a human is lying not ever likely to be completely accurate?

10. What ways have been used in the attempt to improve the accuracy of the testimony of eyewitnesses? What is a cognitive interview?

11. What are three phases of a jury trial in which problems can occur? What are the effects of pretrial publicity on jurors' perceptions of suspects? How can judges and lawyers attempt to remedy the problem of pretrial publicity bias?

12. How do individual jurors process evidence during a trial? In which two orders can lawyers present evidence? Which order is more effective? Given these findings, why may the felony conviction rate in America be as high as it is?

13. What are the benefits of jury deliberations? How are minorities influential in jury deliberation?

14. Why do people obey laws? What explanation does deterrence theory offer? What does this theory fail to explain? Why?

15. What is procedural justice? How important do people consider it to be?

PRACTICE QUIZ SOCIAL PSYCHOLOGY IN ACTION 3

Fill-in-the-Blank

1. The process by which people notice and pay attention to a subset of information available in the environment is called _____.

2. The process by which people store in memory information they have acquired from the environment is called _____.

3. The process by which people recall information stored in their memories is called _____.

4. The process where memory for an event becomes distorted by information that is encountered after the event has occurred is called _____.

5. The process whereby people try to identify the sources of their memories is called

_____.

6. A machine used in lie detection that measures people's physiological responses while they answer questions is called a(n) _____.

7. The finding that people are better at recognising faces of their own race compared to other races is called _____.

8. A technique which attempts to increase the accuracy of eyewitness testimony by directing attention to details of the crime is called the _____.

9. The belief that harsh penalties keep people from breaking laws is the major tenet of

_____.

10. People's judgements as to the fairness of the legal system is called _____.

Multiple Choice

11. Lindsay et al. (1981) found that participants who viewed the videotaped cross-examination of an eyewitness to a staged calculator theft
    a) overestimated the accuracy of eyewitnesses.
    b) did not rely heavily on eyewitness testimony.
    c) allowed their biases to distort the testimony of eyewitnesses.
    d) made source misattributions regarding the eyewitness.

12. It is very likely that witnesses to real crimes will give inaccurate testimony because
    a) eyewitnesses feel that criminals will seek revenge for testimony that convicts them.
    b) emotions experienced while witnessing the crime will be evoked during testimony and interfere with recall.
    c) crimes usually occur under the very conditions that make acquisition difficult.
    d) arousal interferes with the storage of memories.

13. A cognitive process where memory for an event becomes distorted by information that is encountered after the event occurs is called
    a) acquisition.
    b) storage.
    c) retrieval.
    d) reconstructive memory.

14. Lindsay and Wells (1985) found that witnesses were less likely to identify an innocent individual as a criminal when they viewed pictures of people presented
    a) simultaneously.
    b) sequentially.
    c) repeatedly.
    d) on a single occasion.

15. Someone who is motivated to tell a lie
    a) is likely to be caught by anyone.
    b) will be unable to conceal the lie as well as someone who lies casually.
    c) can usually get away with it.
    d) is likely to be caught only by experts in lie detection.

16. Which of the following influences are likely to lead juries to reach unfair verdicts?
    a) biased pretrial publicity
    b) faulty information processing during the trial
    c) normative influence during deliberation
    d) all of the above

17. Since jurors decide upon a "best story" to explain the evidence, a good lawyer would present her witnesses
    a) in order of ascending credibility.
    b) in order of descending credibility.
    c) in an manner which reveals the order of the events as they occurred.
    d) in a manner which leads to a startling and dramatic revelation.

18. Jurors tend to put a lot of faith in eyewitness testimony because
    a) eyewitnesses are in a position of high status in the courtroom.
    b) jurors have a natural bias toward conviction.
    c) normative pressures to side with the eyewitness are high in the courtroom.
    d) they assume that the witness's confidence is a good indicator of accuracy.

19. Retrieval is the process by which people
    a) notice and pay attention to a subset of information available in the environment.
    b) store information in memory that they have acquired from the environment.
    c) rehearse information so that it will not be immediately forgotten.
    d) recall information that is stored in their memories.

20. Why are people likely to give inaccurate accounts of events when asked misleading questions?
    a) because the questions change what people are willing to report
    b) because people assume that the misinformation presented in the question came from their own memories
    c) because the misinformation presented in the question conflicts with stored information and produces dissonance
    d) because the questions bias acquisition

21. Pretrial publicity tends to bias jurors in favour of "guilty" verdicts if the publicity
    a)   arouses public passions.
    b)   evokes counterargumentation by prospective jurors.
    c)   is presented in a factual manner.
    d)   frustrates prospective jurors trying to form an unbiased opinion.

22. Though the media qualifies incriminating statements with words like "allegedly," such statements bias readers because
    a)   mere exposure to the name of the accused increases liking for the individual.
    b)   readers envy the status given to people whose name appears in the paper.
    c)   readers associate the name of the accused with the crime.
    d)   people have a difficult time processing qualifiers while they read.

23. The presence of minority opposition in a jury increases the likelihood that
    a)   a guilty verdict will be rendered.
    b)   the facts in the case will be carefully considered.
    c)   self-awareness among jurors will be high.
    d)   a not guilty verdict will be rendered.

24. According to your text, which of the following has been used to increase the accuracy of eyewitness testimony?
    a)   the cognitive interview
    b)   exposure to pretrial publicity
    c)   memory enhancing drugs
    d)   inducing belief in the just world hypothesis

Short Essay

25. As a social psychologist, you have been contracted by a defence attorney to give your expert opinion on eyewitness accuracy following testimony by a woman who swears that she saw the defendant murder someone. What would you tell the court?

26. If juries usually stick with the verdict favoured by the initial majority of jurors, why should we insist that juries deliberate until they reach consensus on that verdict?

27. Describe the three stages of memory processing that an eyewitness must successfully complete in order to give accurate testimony.

28. Describe legal procedures aimed at eliminating biases created by pretrial publicity. Why are some of these procedures less than perfect remedies?

29. What reasons exist to explain why people obey the law? What are aspects of the legal system that help keep people from committing crimes?

ANSWER SECTION

CHAPTER 1: INTRODUCTION TO SOCIAL PSYCHOLOGY

Answer Key

Fill-in-the-blank

1.   social psychology (p. 4)
2.   social influence (p. 4)
3.   construal (p. 4)
4.   sociology (p. 8)
5.   individual differences (p. 9)
6.   personality psychology (p. 9)
7.   the fundamental attribution error (p. 10)
8.   Behaviourism (p. 13)
9.   Gestalt psychology (p. 14)
10.   self-esteem (p. 17)
11.   social cognition (p. 20)
12.   self-fulfilling prophecy (p. 21)

Multiple Choice:

13.   A (p. 4)
14.   C (p. 5)
15.   A (p. 9)
16.   C (p. 10)
17.   A (p. 13)
18.   A (p. 18)
19.   D (p. 20)
20.   A (p. 4)
21.   A (p. 8)
22.   A (p. 10)
23.   D (p. 14)
24.   D (p. 20)
25.   B (p. 20)
26.   D (p. 21)
27.   C (p. 23)

Short Essay

28.   Linda is most likely to identify psychological processes, like frustration, that produce aggression. Mark is likely to identify broad societal factors, like social class, that may affect aggression. (p. 8)

29.   The self-esteem approach assumes that behaviour is motivated by the desire to perceive ourselves favourably and that we may place a slightly different spin on reality to achieve this end. The social cognition approach assumes that we want to perceive the world accurately but that several obstacles may block this goal. (pp. 17-22)

30. Social psychology takes a scientific approach to the study of human behaviour which allows it to explain the causes of behaviour and demonstrate the conditions under which (sometimes opposite) behaviours will occur. (pp. 5-7)

31. Your example should reflect how an expectancy actually caused a change in your social environment so that your expectancy was confirmed. Expecting it to rain and finding that it does rain, for instance, is not an example of the self-fulfilling prophesy because you did not cause it to rain. (pp. 21-22)

32. Your essay should include instances of how pervasive social influence is and how we are not always aware of how it changes our behaviour. (pp. 3-5)

CHAPTER 2: METHODOLOGY: HOW SOCIAL PSYCHOLOGISTS DO RESEARCH

Answer Key

Fill-in-the-Blank

1.   participant observation (p. 36)
2.   archival analysis (p. 37)
3.   interjudge reliability (p. 37)
4.   correlational method (p. 39)
5.   correlation coefficient (p. 39)
6.   random selection (p. 40)
7.   experimental method (p. 44)
8.   independent variable (p. 47)
9.   dependent variable (p. 47)
10.   internal validity (p. 48)
11.   random assignment to condition (p. 48)
12.   probability level (p. 48)
13.   external validity (p. 49)
14.   psychological realism (p. 50)
15.   replication (p. 51)
16.   meta analysis (p. 51)
17.   field experiment (p. 53)
18.   applied research (p. 58)
19.   informed consent (p. 55)
20.   deception (p. 55)
21.   debriefing (p. 56)

Multiple Choice:

22.   B (p. 33)
23.   D (p. 37)
24.   B (p. 39)
25.   A (p. 40)
26.   D (p. 42)
27.   B (p. 53)
28.   A (p. 51)
29.   C (p. 51)
30.   A (p. 37)
31.   B (p. 39)
32.   B (p. 47)
33.   A (p. 49)
34.   D (p. 49)
35.   B (p. 49)
36.   A (p. 54)
37.   B (p. 58)

38. Common public behaviours are assessed by unobtrusive systematic observation. Behaviours not observable to "outsiders" are assessed by participant observation. Behaviours that change over time or across different cultures are assessed by archival analysis. (pp. 35-37)

39. You cannot generalise survey results to a population that is not represented by your sample. Members of the community who watch other local news programs, who were not home on this particular night, or who were unwilling to call the station are not represented here. (pp. 40-42)

40. Anything in addition to the independent variable that varies could also have caused your results to turn out the way they did. Therefore, the exact cause of your results cannot be known. (pp. 47-49)

41. The setting of highly controlled experiments is often artificial. Results from such experiments may not generalise to everyday life. By replicating the experiment in the field, this limitation can be overcome. (pp. 49-52)

42. Ethical guidelines tell us deception may be used only if no other means of testing the hypothesis is available and only if an Institutional Review Board rules that the experiment does not put participants at undo risk. Following the deception experiment, participants must be provided with a full description and explanation of all procedures including the necessity of deception. (pp. 55-56)

CHAPTER 3: SOCIAL COGNITION: HOW WE THINK ABOUT THE SOCIAL WORLD

Answer Key

Fill-in-the-blank

1.   schemas (p. 63)
2.   counterfactual thinking (p. 90)
3.   perseverance effect (p. 71)
4.   self-fulfilling prophecy (p. 71)
5.   judgmental heuristic (p. 76)
6.   availability heuristic (p. 77)
7.   representativeness heuristic (p. 80)
8.   base rate information (p. 80)
9.   anchoring/adjustment heuristic (p. 81)
10. biased sampling (p. 82)
11. overconfidence barrier (p. 94)
12. accessibility (p. 67)
13. priming (p. 68)
14. automatic processing (p. 85)

Multiple Choice:

15. C (p. 64)
16. B (p. 71)
17. B (p. 71)
18. A (p. 77)
19. D (p. 80)
20. B (p. 85)
21. D (p. 94)
22. D (p. 66)
23. B (p. 65)
24. D (p. 71)
25. B (p. 80)
26. A (p. 90)
27. B (p. 85)
28. B (p. 89)
29. A (p. 92)

Short Essay

30.   Judgements are based on the ease with which something can be brought to mind when the availability heuristic is used. Things are classified according to how similar they are to a "typical" case when the representativeness heuristic is used. Judgements are made by adjusting an answer away from an initial value when the anchoring/adjustment heuristic is used. (pp. 76-85)

31. Asking people to consider the opposite point of view to their own makes people realise that there are other ways to construe the world. The effectiveness of this approach suggests that overconfidence results from people noticing, interpreting, and remembering only information that is consistent with their particular schemas. (p. 94)

32. Cultures determine what schemas we learn and remember. What is valued in a particular culture is more likely to be a part of a well-developed schema. (pp. 73-75)

33. Automatic processing requires less mental effort than does controlled processing. Automatic processing is nonconscious while controlled processing requires conscious awareness. Thought suppression requires the cooperation of both automatic and controlled processing. Automatic processing searches for the unwanted thought and controlled processing is used to think about something else when the thought is present. (pp. 83-87)

34. Amy's counting on people's tendency to insufficiently adjust their estimates away from an anchor when they use the adjustment/anchoring heuristic to decide how much they'll offer for the car. (pp. 81-85)

35. Your attempts at correcting your friend's errors of inference should be aimed at reducing his/her overconfidence (first by overcoming the overconfidence barrier), by asking him/her to consider the opposite point of view, and by recommending college statistics courses, one-time lessons in reasoning, or training in research design. (pp. 94-95)

CHAPTER 4: SOCIAL PERCEPTION: HOW WE COME TO UNDERSTAND OTHER PEOPLE

Answer Key

Fill-in-the-Blank

1.   social perception (p. 100)
2.   nonverbal communication (p. 100)
3.   encode, decode (p. 101)
4.   display rules   (p. 105)
5.   affect blends (p. 105)
6.   emblems   (p. 108)
7.   implicit personality theories (p. 108)
8.   attribution theory (p. 111)
9.   internal attribution (p. 111)
10.   external attribution (p. 111)
11.   covariation model (p. 113)
12.   consensus information (p. 113)
13.   distinctiveness information (p. 113)
14.   consistency information (p. 113)
15.   fundamental attribution error (p. 116)
16.   actor/observer difference (p. 121)
17.   self-serving attributions (p. 124)
18.   unrealistic optimism (p. 127)
19.   belief in a just world (p. 132)

Multiple Choice

20.   C (p. 111)
21.   C (p. 121)
22.   A (p. 132)
23.   D (p. 100)
24.   A (p. 105)
25.   C (p. 108)
26.   D (p. 105)
27.   B (p. 111)
28.   D (p. 113)
29.   B (p. 121)
30.   C (p. 134)
31.   A (p. 134)

32.   Your example should depict an internal attribution for a recent success and an external attribution for a recent failure. (pp. 124-127)

33.   You should discuss blaming the victim as by-product of how we make attributions for the causes of the behaviour of others. You might mention how we decide that the victim should have done something to avoid or to control the outcome even if it was not possible to do so. The belief in a just world might also be cited as a foundation for blaming the victim. (pp. 129-133)

34.   The fundamental attribution error is the tendency to attribute the behaviour of others to factors internal to them and to ignore the role of the situation as a cause for much human behaviour. For example, a police officer is required by law to enforce traffic regulations, but we might see such behaviour as the product of the officer's personality. You should make mention of how the person and their personality is far more salient than situational factors in most circumstances, and that this saliency contributes to the fundamental attribution error. You might also note the role of culture in the fundamental attribution error. (pp. 115-121)

CHAPTER 5: SELF-KNOWLEDGE: HOW WE COME TO UNDERSTAND OURSELVES

Answer Key

Fill-in-the-Blank

1.   self-concept (p. 140)
2.   introspection (p. 148)
3.   self-awareness theory (p. 149)
4.   causal theory (p. 153)
5.   self-perception theory (p. 155)
6.   intrinsic motivation (p. 155)
7.   overjustification effect (p. 156)
8.   two-factor theory of emotion (p. 160)
9.   misattribution of arousal (p. 162)
10.   looking glass self (p. 165)
11.   social comparison theory (p. 167)
12.   upward social comparison (p. 169)
13.   self-presentation (p. 171)
14.   impression management (p. 171)

Multiple Choice:

15.   A (p. 141)
16.   C (p. 144)
17.   D (p. 154)
18.   D (p. 155)
19.   A (p. 155)
20.   B (p. 156)
21.   B (p. 157)
22.   C (p. 160)
23.   B (p. 162)
24.   D (p. 165)
25.   C (p. 167)
26.   D (p. 148)
27.   B (p. 153)
28.   D (p. 156)
29.   B (p. 160)
30.   C (p. 163)
31.   A (p. 165)
32.   A (p. 168)

33.   According to self-perception theory, when the causes of our behaviour are ambiguous, we are in functionally the same role as an outside observer attributing our own behaviour to our attitudes and traits (note that these are therefore internal attributions). (p. 155)

34.   As you introspect about the reasons why you are attracted to your recent dating partner, you are likely to bring to mind reasons that sound plausible and are available but which may not be the actual reasons. A negative consequence of identifying the wrong reasons is that you may change your mind about how you feel to match those reasons. For instance, if you decide that you are attracted to someone because the two of you share a common hobby, you may decide that such a reason is not justification for pursuing a relationship and lose interest. (p. 148)

35.   When we're self-aware, we form more accurate judgements of ourselves and may behave in a manner more consistent with our internal values and standards. However, self-awareness is uncomfortable and may cause us to engage in deleterious behaviours such as drinking alcohol etc. to avoid self-awareness when we cannot change our behaviours. (pp. 148-152)

36.   Both theories maintain that we come to understand ourselves by observing our own behaviour and finding an appropriate explanation. The theories differ in two ways. First, each explains how we come to know a different feature of ourselves. Self-perception theory explains how we know what we think and what kind of person we are. The two-factor theory explains how we know how we feel. Second, each theory claims we use a different type of behaviour to achieve self-understanding. Self-perception theory says we make internal attributions from observing overt behaviour. The two factor theory states we label behaviour that is associated with physiological arousal. (pp. 155-162)

37.   Before your pay raise there were no large extrinsic rewards for working at the library. When asked, therefore, you are more likely to conclude that you work there because you like it. If you overjustify your reason for working there after your pay raise, the conspicuous external reward will grab your attention, cause you to discount the role of your intrinsic interest in the job, and lead you to conclude that you like the job less. (pp. 156-160)

38.   The looking glass self is the self we see when we adopt another person's perspective from which to view ourselves. It is constructed as we adopt, over time, such a perspective. Research demonstrating that apes raised in isolation did not recognise themselves in a mirror suggests that social interaction is necessary for the development of the self. (pp. 165-166)

CHAPTER 6: SELF-JUSTIFICATION AND THE NEED TO MAINTAIN SELF-ESTEEM

Answer Key

Fill-in-the-Blank

1. cognitive dissonance (p. 192)
2. post-decision dissonance (p. 195)
3. justification of effort (p. 199)
4. external justification (p. 201)
5. internal justification (p. 201)
6. counter-attitudinal advocacy (p. 201)
7. insufficient punishment (p. 204)
8. self-affirmation theory (p. 184)
9. self-verification theory (p. 190)
10. rationalization trap (p. 211)
11. self-justification (p. 205)
12. self-discrepancy theory (p. 178)
13. counter-attitudinal advocacy (p. 201)

Multiple Choice:

14. B (p. 194)
15. D (p. 195)
16. C (p. 198)
17. C (p. 201)
18. B (p. 208)
19. A (p. 181)
20. C (p. 191)
21. D (p. 213)
22. B (p. 198)
23. D (p. 196)
24. A (p. 201)
25. C (p. 205)
26. B (p. 206)
27. B (p. 207)
28. A (p. 184)
29. B (p. 211)

30. Members will justify their efforts to join the group and will find the group attractive even if the group turns out to have little to offer. (pp. 198-201)

31. $100 is sufficient external justification for claiming loyalty to any radio station but a T-shirt is insufficient justification that will motivate a search for internal justification and a will result in a more favourable evaluation of the radio station. (pp. 178-180)

32. If writing the essay caused physiological arousal then participants who believed they should be feeling relaxed felt this arousal and assumed that it would have been greater still had they not taken the drug. If arousal motivates attitude change then participants believing that they are highly aroused should have been especially motivated to change their attitudes. Greater attitude change among subjects who'd taken the relaxing placebo supports these claims. (pp. 206-207)

33. Cognitive dissonance theory maintains that we reduce dissonance by changing behaviours or by adding or changing cognitions to justify behaviours. Self-evaluation maintenance theory states that we reduce dissonance by improving our performance relative to our friend's, distancing ourselves from the individual, or by reducing how relevant the task is to our self-image. Self-affirmation theory asserts that we reduce dissonance by affirming our competence and integrity in an unrelated area where our esteem is not threatened. (pp. 181-192)

CHAPTER 7: ATTITUDES AND ATTITUDE CHANGE: INFLUENCING THOUGHTS AND FEELINGS

Answer Key

Fill-in-the-blank

1.   attitude (p. 220)
2.   affective (p. 221)
3.   cognitive (p. 221)
4.   behavioural (p. 221)
5.   Yale Attitude Change Approach (p. 237)
6.   Elaboration Likelihood Model (p. 238)
7.   central (p. 239)
8.   peripheral (p. 239)
9.   fear-arousing communication (p. 246)
10.   cognitively based attitudes (p. 221)
11.   affectively based attitudes (p. 221)
12.   classical conditioning (p. 222)
13.   operant conditioning (p. 222)
14.   behaviourally based attitudes (p. 223)
15.   attitude accessibility (p. 226)
16.   attitude inoculation (p. 253)
17.   reactance theory (p. 256)
18.   theory of planned behaviour (p. 230)
19.   subjective norms (p. 231)
20.   subliminal messages (p. 250)

Multiple Choice:

21.   C (p. 221)
22.   A (p. 236)
23.   B (p. 242)
24.   D (p. 246)
25.   C (p. 222)
26.   D (p. 241)
27.   C (p. 244)
28.   B (p. 250)
29.   D (p. 230)
30.   B (p. 238)
31.   D (p. 245)
32.   B (p. 226)
33.   C (p. 256)
34.   D (p. 230)

35. Your example should indicate that a cognitively based attitude is founded on people's beliefs about the properties of the attitude object, that an affectively based attitude is founded on people's emotions and values that are evoked by the attitude object, and that a behaviourally based attitude is derived from people's observations of how they behave toward the attitude object. (pp. 221-225)

36. Persuasive attempts "boomerang," or cause an increased interest in the activity your persuasive attempt is aimed at discouraging, when strong prohibitions for engaging in the activity are used. In part, this occurs because, according to reactance theory, we are motivated to restore a sense of freedom when we perceive that we are not free to engage in the activity. On means of restoring a sense of freedom is to perform the behaviour. The boomerang effect also occurs because strong prohibitions provide ample and conspicuous external justification for not engaging in the behaviour. Under such conditions, overjustification is likely to occur. That is, people will underestimate the intrinsic reasons for avoiding the behaviour and come to believe that they enjoy the activity more. (p. 256)

37. People's attitudes toward greeting cards are clearly affectively based. Your approach should therefore be to play on these emotions. You would recommend presenting ads that depict joyous birthdays and weddings, proud moments like graduation etc. (pp. 247-249)

38. According to the Elaboration Likelihood Model, people take the central route to persuasion when they are both motivated and able to attend to arguments presented. Subsequent attitude change will persist, be consistent with behaviours, and resist counterpersuasion. If people are either unmotivated or unable to attend to the arguments, they will attend to cues which are peripheral to the message itself and take the peripheral route to persuasion. Subsequent attitude change will be short-lived, be inconsistent with behaviours, and will change again in the face of counterpersuasion. (pp. 238-245)

39. Attitude inoculation makes people immune to attempts to change cognitively based attitudes by initially exposing them to small doses of the arguments against their position. Peer pressure is likely to play on adolescents' feelings of autonomy and social rejection. That is, it is directed at changing affectively, rather than cognitively based attitudes. The attitude inoculation technique can be modified by exposing adolescents to small doses of peer pressure during role-playing interventions. (pp. 253-255)

CHAPTER 8: CONFORMITY: INFLUENCING BEHAVIOUR

Answer Key

Fill-in-the-Blank

1.   conformity (p. 261)
2.   informational social influence (p. 262)
3.   private acceptance (p. 264)
4.   public compliance   (p. 264)
5.   contagion (p. 265)
6   social norms (p. 270)
7.   normative social influence (p. 270)
8.   door-in-the-face technique (p. 287)
9.   reciprocity norm (p. 288)
10.   social impact theory (p. 274)
11.   idiosyncrasy credits (p. 282)
12.   minority influence (p. 286)
13.   foot in the door technique (p. 289)

Multiple Choice:

14.   A (p. 263)
15.   A (p. 268)
16.   B (p. 271)
17.   C (p. 274)
18.   D (p. 288)
19.   D (p. 274)
20.   C (p. 280)
21.   B (p. 279)
22.   D (p. 280)
23.   D (p. 296)
24.   C (p. 297)
25.   D (p. 261)
26.   B (p. 264)
27.   C (p. 272)
28.   A (p. 274)
29.   A (p. 278)
30.   D (p. 279)
31.   B (p. 288)
32.   C (p. 297)

33.   Participants complied to normative pressures to please the experimenter, used the experimenter as an expert source of information in an ambiguous situation, and got caught in a web of conflicting social norms that led them to follow an inappropriate "obey authority" norm.
(pp. 296-299)

34.   Informational Social Influence   Normative Social Influence
       Sherif   Asch
       Milgram   Schachter
       minority influence   Milgram
       contagion
       (pp. 262-299)

35.   Both forms of influence produce conformity to the behaviours of others. Informational social influence, which produces private acceptance, is motivated by the need to be right while normative social influence, which produces public compliance, is motivated by the need to be liked. (pp. 296-298)

36.   The unambiguous nature of Asch's line matching task required that participants blindly conform in order to go along. The demonstration is all the more dramatic because participants conformed in order to be liked by a group of strangers. (pp. 271-274)

37.   According to social impact theory the impact that a group will have on an individual is a function of the group's strength, or how important the group is to the individual, its immediacy, how close the group is to the individual in space and time during the influence attempt, and it's number, the size of the group. (pp. 274-280)

CHAPTER 9: GROUP PROCESSES: INFLUENCE IN SOCIAL GROUPS

Answer Key

Fill-in-the-Blank

1. social facilitation (p. 312)
2. social loafing (p. 315)
3. deindividuation (p. 318)
4. process loss (p. 320)
5. groupthink (p. 323)
6. group polarization (p. 326)
7. contingency theory of leadership (p. 330)
8. relationship-oriented leader (p. 330)
9. great person theory (p. 327)
10. tit-for-tat (p. 335)
11. negotiation (p. 338)
12. integrative solution (p. 339)
13. transactive memory (p. 322)
14. social dilemma (p. 333)

Multiple Choice:

15. C (p. 313)
16. B (p. 315)
17. B (p. 312)
18. D (p. 326)
19. A (p. 339)
20. B (p. 311)
21. A (p. 312)
22. B (p. 333)
23. C (p. 318)
24. C (p. 327)
25. D (p. 330)
26. A (p. 327)
27. D (p. 335)
28. B (p. 318)
29. A (p. 321)
30. B (p. 337)

Short Essay

31. Group polarization is the tendency for groups to make decisions that are more extreme than the initial inclinations of its members. According to a persuasive arguments interpretation of group polarization, the phenomenon results because members present strong and novel arguments in support of their initial recommendation to the group during discussion. According to a motivational interpretation, discussion serves to reveal the recommendation that is favoured by the group. In order to be liked by the group, members then adopt a recommendation similar to everyone else's but a little more extreme. (pp. 325-327)

32. Deindividuation loosens constraints on behaviours when crowds make members less accountable for their actions and foster anonymity. Add to this a situation that presents negative cues, and inhibitions against negative behaviours will be decreased. Negative behaviour will ensue.
(pp. 317-320)

33. Groupthink occurs when certain preconditions are met, such as when the group is highly cohesive, is isolated from contrary opinion, and is ruled by a directive leader. Symptoms of groupthink include feelings of invulnerability, self-censorship, direct pressures on dissenters to conform, and an illusion of unanimity. Groupthink prevents groups from considering the full range of alternative available to them, from developing contingency plans, and from considering the risks of the preferred choice. (pp. 323-325)

34. Negotiation is a form of communication between opposing sides in a conflict in which the parties make offers and counteroffers, and where a solution occurs only when both parties agree. Two strategies that groups communicating with one another can use are to make concessions and to look for integrative solutions, solutions to a conflict that find outcomes favourable to both sides. When negotiations break down because the two sides refuse to communicate, a neutral third party may be called on to mediate or arbitrate. Mediators allow the opposing parties to resolve their conflict by making suggestions and by searching for agreeable solutions. Arbitrators impose a decision on the parties after hearing arguments on both sides. (pp. 338-340)

CHAPTER 10: INTERPERSONAL ATTRACTION: FROM FIRST IMPRESSIONS TO CLOSE RELATIONSHIPS

Answer Key

Fill-in-the-Blank

1. propinquity effect (p. 347)
2. mere exposure effect (p. 348)
3. love styles (p. 362)
4. social exchange (p. 372
5. comparison level (p. 373
6. comparison level for alternatives (p. 373)
7. equity (p. 373)
8. companionate love (p. 360)
9. passionate love (p. 360)
10. triangular theory of love (p. 361)
11. investment model (p. 375)
12. exchange (p. 376)
13. communal (p. 376)
14. attachment styles (p. 369)
15. secure (p. 369)
16. avoidant (p. 369)
17. anxious/ambivalent (p. 369)
18. commitment calibration (p. 378)

Multiple Choice:

19. D (p. 347)
20. A (p. 352)
21. B (p. 354)
22. D (p. 372)
23. A (p. 373)
24. B (p. 362)
25. D (p. 375)
26. C (p. 376)
27. C (p. 363)
28. B (p. 350)
29. D (p. 373)
30. A (p. 377)
31. D (p. 369)
32. C (p. 369)
33. D (p. 369)
34. D (p. 363)
35. A (p. 369)
36. B (p. 378)

Short Essay

37. We develop favourable impressions of individuals when repeated exposure owing to propinquity makes the person familiar. We like individuals whose characteristics and beliefs are similar to our own. We like people who offer praise so long as it seems sincere. We like people who like us, especially if we have gained in their positive estimation of us. Finally, good looks can increase interpersonal attraction. (pp. 347-353)

38. The facial features associated with the attractiveness of females include: large eyes, a small nose, a small chin, prominent cheekbones, and a big smile. The features associated with the attractiveness in males include: large eyes, prominent cheekbones, a large chin, and a big smile. Assumptions people make about attractive versus less attractive people include: they are more successful, intelligent, adjusted, exciting, and socially competent. A consequence of making such assumptions is that due to the self-fulfilling prophecy, we may behave in ways that confirm our expectations about attractive people. (pp. 353-359)

39. Attachment theory assumes that attachment styles that we learn as infants and young children generalise to all of our relationships with others. Infants with responsive caregivers develop a secure attachment style and are able to develop mature, stable relationships later in life. Infants with aloof and distant caregivers develop an avoidant style are untrusting and find it difficult to develop intimacy. Infants whose caregivers are inconsistent and overbearing in their affections develop an anxious\ambivalent style. These individuals desire intimacy but fear that their affections will not be returned. (pp. 368-372)

40. The six styles of love are ludus (love is a game), Eros (passionate love), storge (friendship love), mania (emotional love), agape (selfless love), and pragma (pragmatic love). (pp. 362-363)

41. Both theories claim that perceived rewards and punishments in a relationship determine relationship satisfaction. Equity theory claims that the notion of fairness or equity is additionally important. According to equity theory, even if the rewards of both partners outweigh the costs, the relationship will be unsatisfying if it is inequitable. (pp. 372-377)

CHAPTER 11: PROSOCIAL BEHAVIOUR: WHY DO PEOPLE HELP?

Answer Key

Fill-in-the-Blank

1.   prosocial behaviour (p. 389)
2.   altruism (p. 389)
3.   kin selection (p. 390)
4.   norm of reciprocity (p. 392)
5.   evolutionary psychology (p. 390)
6.   empathy (p. 395)
7.   empathy-altruism hypothesis (p. 395)
8.   altruistic personality (p. 399)
9.   in-group (p. 404)
10.   negative-state relief hypothesis (p. 402)
11.   urban-overload hypothesis (p. 405)
12.   bystander effect (p. 408)
13.   pluralistic ignorance (p. 410)
14.   diffusion of responsibility (p. 411)

Multiple Choice

15.   C (p. 389)
16.   A (p. 390)
17.   B (p. 393)
18.   D (p. 395)
19.   D (p. 402)
20.   C (p. 404)
21.   C (p. 400)
22.   B (p. 402)
23.   B (p. 408)
24.   B (p. 411)
25.   C (p. 119)
26.   A (p. 390)
27.   A (p. 416)
28.   B (p. 400)
29.   A (p. 402)
30.   C (p. 405)
31.   A (p. 407)
32.   D (p. 414)
33.   C (p. 412)

34. According to social exchange theory, we will help others when the rewards of helping outweigh the costs. In this situation, the rewards, such as the esteem of others at the concert and self-esteem must have outweighed the costs. Costs include the potential embarrassment of attempting to help someone who, in fact, was not ill and the possibility that you yourself might get hurt. (pp. 393-394)

35. Prosocial behaviour is performed with the goal of benefiting another. It may or may not be performed without any regard to self-interests. Altruistic behaviour is performed with the goal of benefiting others without any regard to self-interests. Hence, all altruistic acts are prosocial, but not all prosocial acts may be altruistic. (p. 389)

36. 1) get people's attention so that they will notice that there is a potential problem, 2) indicate that you are indeed hurt and need assistance, 3) single someone out by making eye contact and addressing the person so that he or she feels that the responsibility is his or hers alone, 4) suggest an appropriate form of assistance, and 5) ensure that the person implements the assistance by reassuring the person that you would be greatly appreciative of his or her help. (pp. 406-413)

37. By reducing the stimulation people encounter, helping can be increased. You may not be able to reduce the population of a city but as an architect you might be able to design buildings that limit the amount of unwanted contact people experience. Likewise, though you might not be able to reduce the number of bystanders present in emergency situations, you can instruct people on the causes of bystander intervention. Research has shown that such instruction increases prosocial behaviour. (pp. 416-420)

38. According to the sociobiological approach, we are motivated to help others when helping increases the likelihood that our genes will live on in subsequent generations. Social exchange theory maintains that we help when the rewards of doing so outweigh the costs. The empathy-altruism hypothesis states that when we feel empathy for another person, altruistic concerns for that person motivate helping without any concern for ourselves. (pp. 390-399)

39. According to the negative-state relief hypothesis, we help people in order to relieve our own sadness and distress. Given that you believe that your negative state will be prolonged by the drug you have just taken, helping in this situation will not make you feel any better. The negative-state relief hypothesis therefore predicts that you will not help. (pp. 400-402)

CHAPTER 12: AGGRESSION: WHY WE HURT OTHER PEOPLE

Answer Key

Fill-in-the-Blank

1.   aggression (p. 425)
2.   hostile aggression (p. 425)
3.   instrumental aggression (p. 425)
4.   Eros (p. 426)
5.   Thanatos (p. 426)
6.   amygdala   (p. 429)
7.   testosterone (p. 429)
8.   frustration-aggression theory (p. 435)
9.   relative deprivation (p. 436)
10.   aggressive stimulus (p. 439)
11.   social learning theory (p. 441)
12.   catharsis (p. 454)

Multiple Choice:

13.   D (p. 425)
14.   C (p. 429)
15.   B (p. 429)
16.   A (p. 434)
17.   C (p. 440)
18.   C (p. 444)
19.   C (p. 451)
20.   A (p. 454)
21.   A (p. 456)
22.   D (p. 458)
23.   C (p. 460)
24.   B (p. 426)
25.   A (p. 426)
26.   B (p. 429)
27.   C (p. 435)
28.   D (p. 436)
29.   A (p. 441)
30.   B (p. 448)
31.   B (p. 459)
32.   A (p. 462)

33.   Cultures vary widely in their degree of aggressiveness. For instance, "primitive" tribes in Central Africa and New Guinea are far less aggressive than our "civilised" modern world. Moreover, there is evidence of changes in the aggression within a culture over time. The Iroquois Indians were peaceful until the European influence brought them into economic competition with neighbouring tribes. (pp. 427-429)

34.   Berkowitz and LePage (1967) have demonstrated increased aggression by angered individuals in the presence of an aggressive stimulus (a gun) and concluded that the "trigger can also pull the finger" of individuals ready to aggress and who have no strong inhibitions against doing so. (pp. 439-441)

35.   Children exposed to a steady diet of violent television are more likely to behave aggressively even if they are not disposed to such behaviour. Additionally, children who watch a lot of violence on TV are less sensitive to subsequent violence they observe. The effects of viewing television violence on aggressive behaviour are similar for adults. (pp. 442-448)

36.   Frustration is the feeling that you are being prevented from obtaining a goal. According to the frustration-aggression theory, frustration produces anger or annoyance and a readiness to aggress. Likelihood of aggressive behaviour depends on: (1) how frustrated you are (frustration increases the closer the goal is), and (2) situational factors conducive to aggressive behaviour (e.g., the victim's inability to retaliate, perception that the frustration is illegitimate, presence of an aggressive stimulus). (pp. 435-437)

37.   The most effective means to reduce your own aggression when you are angry is to avoid engaging in aggressive behaviour. Instead, express your anger calmly. To defuse aggression in someone who you have frustrated, apologise for your behaviour. People can be taught nonaggressive behaviour by imposing swift yet mild punishment, by exposing people to nonaggressive models and by reinforcing their nonaggressive communication and problem-solving behaviours. Finally, by building empathy in people, they are less likely to dehumanise individuals and behave aggressively toward them. (pp. 458-463)

CHAPTER 13: PREJUDICE: CAUSES AND CURES

Answer Key

Fill-in-the-Blank

1.   prejudice (p. 471)
2.   stereotype   (p. 472)
3.   discrimination (p. 473)
4.   out-group homogeneity (p. 481)
5.   bookkeeping (p. 510)
6.   conversion (p. 510)
7.   subtyping (p. 510)
8.   ultimate attribution error (p. 491)
9.   realistic conflict theory (p. 492)
10.   normative conformity (p. 496)
11.   mutually interdependent (p. 512)
12.   jigsaw classroom (p. 514)
13.   stereotype threat (p. 504)
14.   extended contact hypothesis (p. 516)
15.   meta-stereotypes (p. 487)

Multiple Choice

16.   D (p. 472)
17.   A (p. 472)
18.   D (p. 483)
19.   D (p. 492)
20.   C (p. 471)
21.   A (p. 481)
22.   D (p. 499)
23.   D (p. 512)
24.   A (p. 501)
25.   B (p. 503)
26.   A (p. 475)
27.   B (p. 476)
28.   C (p. 485)
29.   A (p. 489)
30.   B (p. 496)
31.   B (p. 506)
32.   C (p. 516)

Short Essay

33.   According to Devine (1989), stereotypes that we all know come to mind automatically
       when we encounter members of the stereotyped group. People who are low in
       prejudice are likely to suppress or override the stereotype by consciously telling
       themselves that the stereotype is inaccurate and unfair. People who are high in
       prejudice are less likely to entertain such thoughts consciously. Consequently, their
       thinking is more likely to be ruled by the stereotype.
       (pp. 482-488)

34.   The ultimate attribution error is committed when we make dispositional attributions for
       entire groups of people and leads us to expect them to behave in stereotypic ways (for
       instance, lazy or stupid). Such biased expectancies are perpetuated by the self-fulfilling
       prophecy when we interact with out-group members in a manner that elicits behaviour
       which confirms the stereotype. (pp. 491-492)

35.   Making the individual aware of disconfirming evidence that is concentrated in only a
       few members of the categorised group will create a sub-stereotype leaving the original
       stereotype intact (subtyping model). Hence, the best strategy for modifying stereotypic
       beliefs with disconfirming evidence is to make the individual aware that such evidence
       exists in many members of the categorised group (bookkeeping model). (pp. 508-510)

36.   Compared to students in traditional classrooms, students in jigsaw classrooms exhibit
       decreased prejudice and stereotyping, increased liking for groupmates both within and
       across ethnic boundaries, increased liking for school, better performance on objective
       exams, increased self-esteem, intermingling, and empathy. (pp. 513-517)

SOCIAL PSYCHOLOGY IN ACTION 1

SOCIAL PSYCHOLOGY AND HEALTH

Answer Key

Fill-in-the-Blank

1.   stress (p. 524)
2.   perceived control (p. 528)
3.   self-efficacy (p. 532)
4.   learned helplessness (p. 534)
5.   stable attribution (p. 534)
6.   internal attribution (p. 534)
7.   global attribution (p. 534)
8.   coping styles (p. 537)
9.   Type A; Type B (p. 538)
10.   social support (p. 543)
11.   buffering hypothesis (p. 544)

Multiple Choice

12.   D (p. 524)
13.   B (p. 528)
14.   C (p. 529)
15.   A (p. 531)
16.   B (p. 534)
17.   D (p. 538)
18.   D (p. 523)
19.   C (p. 527)
20.   B (p. 531)
21.   B (p. 534)
22.   A (p. 534)
23.   A (p. 537)
24.   D (p. 541)

Short Essay

25.   Stress, which lowers the responsiveness of our immune system and makes us more susceptible to disease, can be reduced by increasing people's sense of control and by getting them to explain negative events in a more optimistic way. Social influence techniques can be used to get people to change their health habits. Cognitive dissonance techniques seem particularly effective in getting people to change intractable, ingrained health habits. (pp. 544-547)

26   Research finds that giving residents a sense of control over their lives increases both happiness and health. As director, you should stress to residents that they have the ability to make decisions about their lives at the home and should present them with options from which they can choose. You must be careful, however, not to repeal these changes once implemented. Research finds that instilling a sense of control and then revoking it has more negative consequences than never instilling it in the first place. (pp. 528-532)

27.   According to learned helplessness theory, depression may result from explaining negative events as due to internal, stable, and global causes. You would recommend that your client adopt an optimistic attributional style and explain negative events with external, unstable, and specific attributions. (pp. 534-537)

SOCIAL PSYCHOLOGY IN ACTION 2

SOCIAL PSYCHOLOGY AND THE ENVIRONMENT

Answer Key

Fill-in-the-Blank

1. density (p. 558)
2. crowding (p. 558)
3. sensory overload (p. 562)
4. injunctive norms (p. 570)
5. descriptive norms (p. 570)

Multiple Choice

6.   B (p. 555)
7.   C (p. 555)
8.   B (p. 558)
9.   A (p. 558)
10. C (p. 564)
11. D (p. 568)
12. C (p. 570)
13. D (p. 571)
14. D (p. 554)
15. A (p. 555)
16. D (p. 557)
17. B (p. 558)
18. A (p. 561)
19. C (p. 564)
20. C (p. 564)
21. A (p. 570)
22. B (p. 570)

Short Essay

23. The failure to conserve water is a classic social dilemma. In large groups, like an entire community, communication between members is an impractical means of resolving the dilemma. It may be possible to send committee members door-to-door, asking people to sign petitions condemning wastefulness while making them mindful of their own wasteful behaviour. Because such dissonance arousing techniques require an initial behaviour (e.g., signing the petition), they may also be of limited use on a large scale. Making selfish behaviour public is likely to be an effective strategy in this case. Your committee might decide, for instance, to publish the names of water gluttons in the local newspapers. (pp. 563-567)

24. You might remind people of socially sanctioned behaviours (evoking injunctive norms) by using the waste can or by displaying anti-littering posters. You could change people's perceptions of people's littering behaviour in the park (changing descriptive norms) by removing the litter. In the long run, evoking injunctive norms is likely to be most effective since the effectiveness of descriptive norms depends on everyone's cooperation. (pp. 570-573)

25. Experimental research has demonstrated that when people are exposed to uncontrollable loud noises that they experience learned helplessness which leads to depression, decreased effort, and difficulty in learning. Field studies demonstrate that children attending noisy schools had higher blood pressure, were more easily distracted, and gave up on difficult problems more easily. Likewise, children living in noisy apartment buildings do more poorly on reading tests.
(pp. 555-558)

26. Communication fosters trust and cooperation among members and allows members to persuade each other that selfless behaviour is in the best interests of all. Communication, however, is a strategy that is necessarily limited to small groups. In larger groups, such as entire communities, nations, etc., making selfish behaviour public evokes normative pressures against such behaviour. Another proven technique is to change the way in which people perceive themselves and their social behaviour by first evoking cognitive dissonance. (pp. 563-567)

SOCIAL PSYCHOLOGY IN ACTION 3

SOCIAL PSYCHOLOGY AND THE LAW

Answer Key

Fill-in-the-Blank

1.   acquisition (p. 581)
2.   storage (p. 581)
3.   retrieval (p. 581)
4.   reconstructive memory (p. 585)
5.   source monitoring (p. 586)
6.   polygraph (p. 593)
7.   own-race bias (p. 584)
8.   cognitive interview (p. 596)
9.   deterrence theory (p. 605)
10.   procedural justice (p. 609)

Multiple Choice:

11.   A (p. 580)
12.   C (p. 583)
13.   D (p. 585)
14.   B (p. 585)
15.   C (p. 593)
16.   D (p. 601)
17.   C (p. 603)
18.   D (p. 589)
19.   D (p. 581)
20.   B (p. 585)
21.   A (p. 601)
22.   C (p. 602)
23.   B (p. 605)
24.   A (p. 596)

Short Essay

25.   You would tell the court that people's heavy reliance on eyewitness testimony should be tempered by the knowledge that they often overestimate the accuracy of such testimony. The problem, you would explain, is that people assume that eyewitness confidence is indicative of accuracy when, in fact, the things that make eyewitnesses confident are not the same things that make them accurate. For instance, viewing conditions that decrease accuracy do not generally decrease confidence. Likewise, rehearsing testimony increases confidence but not accuracy. (pp. 580-592)

26. Requiring unanimity makes the jurors consider the evidence more carefully. Furthermore, while a minority is not likely to reverse the majority's verdict, the minority may change the minds of the majority members regarding how guilty the defendant is. For instance, a majority that maintains the guilt of a murder suspect may agree to second- rather than first-degree murder if influenced by a minority. (pp. 604-605)

27. An eyewitness must first acquire the events witnessed. That is, the eyewitness must notice and pay attention to the events (acquisition). Memory of the information that has been acquired must them be stored (storage). Finally, the information that has been stored must be recalled from memory (retrieval). Eyewitnesses can be inaccurate because of problems at any of these three stages. (pp. 581-589)

28. Less-than-perfect remedies for the tendency to render a guilty verdict after exposure to emotional publicity include *voir dire* and instructions by the judge to disregard. Research indicates that jurors who claim that they have not been influenced by publicity nonetheless render more guilty verdicts when the publicity is emotional. Research also shows that instructions to not think about something often have the opposite effect. For instance, trying NOT to think of a white bear evokes images of a white bear. Another problem with pretrial publicity is that people are likely to form negative impressions of individuals whose name appears in a newspaper title along with a negative stimulus even if the title explicitly denies the association. The remedy to this problem is to permit people to serve on the jury only if they have heard nothing about the case. (pp. 601-602)

29. The reasons used to explain why people obey laws are offered by deterrence theory and procedural justice. Deterrence theory explains obeying the law by focusing on the importance of the threat of punishment. In order for deterrence to be effective, however, punishment must be perceived as severe, certain, and immediate. Procedural justice focuses on how people's judgements about the fairness of the legal system influences whether or not they obey a law. The perceived justness of the law and of legal proceedings are important aspects people consider. (pp. 608-610)